Fibromyalgia: The Secret to Recovery

Talor Sela

Cover painting by Talor Sela

TO MY BELOVED PARENTS, HANNA AND
MORDECHAI KRUP, NOBLE, HONEST AND
PURE AT HEART.

"LOVELY AND PLEASANT IN THEIR LIVES,
AND IN THEIR DEATH THEY WERE NOT
DIVIDED".

THEIR MEMORIAL WEBSITE:
WWW.KRUPSTORY.BLOGSPOT.CO.IL

ACKNOWLEDGMENTS

I thank Our Lord the Creator, for, in his hidden ways, he has led me to discover the kindness that lies within me; to recognize that I and my surroundings are bountiful; to transform my life; to acquire strengths that made me be who I am today; to dream new dreams and fulfill them one by one; to believe and know Him.

I thank my beloved parents, Hana and Mordechai Krup RIP, who raised me with endless love and have been my rock since I can remember, who let me know that as long as they live, I could always depend on them.

I thank my kind children, Alon, Eyal, Ofir and Itay, for having the wisdom to find their own path in life, coupled with their commitment to support me when called upon, and for teaching me throughout the years.

I thank my dear sister, Zipi Kerlitz, who has walked beside me and supported many of the decisions that changed my life.

I thank my brother in-law, Avraham Kerlitz, for pitching in and providing support and advice whenever I asked for it.

I thank my cousin, Israel Galon, for in his unique and extraordinary humane way of treating people, he lent an ear to my cries, provided comfort and prayer in times of need and encouraged me in my journey.

I thank Rafi Yaakobi from the "School of Friendship", who has provided me with an accurate view of my life and made me divert my sorrows towards a path of creativity and ongoing success.

I thank Dina and Yehuda Shmargad, friends of heart and soul, loyal, supportive, attentive and encouraging, who have always been there for me ever since I was young.

I thank Poria and Ever Lavi, who, by day or night, provided me with a crutch on maddening days, stood by me whenever I stumbled and supported me without question while always keeping a positive outlook. The conversations with you always bear fruit, and in your company I feel safe to be who I am, and receive constant backing to go out and accomplish that which is important to me. It is not taken for granted.

I thank Pirchia Rechavi, my children's ultimate nanny. Her dedicated and attentive care of my children and my own needs has made it easier for me to raise them and she has played a great part in making their childhood memories full of safety, belongingness, warmth and love.

I thank Michal Cohen, my devoted friend, who treated my body and my soul in times of need, which were plenty.

I thank Lizzy Zommer, who has been the first and only one who gave voice to the words, "Fibromyalgia can be cured. It is possible to make it through," in my presence. With that, she has planted in me the knowledge and will to pursue my health and find my own path. She has given her time and attention in order to encourage my every action and has been an inspiration and hope to me.

I thank Selvi Peled, for supporting, encouraging and guiding in the right place, at the right time.

I thank my friend, Daniela Aviv, who from the first moment we met, bestowed warmth upon me, encouraged me to go out and live, taught me how to broaden my social circle, never gave up on me when I was down, and kept me safe so that I could go with the flow of life.

I thank my spiritual teachers whom I have met on my journey, for providing light to my darkness, and many others I met on my voyage: therapists, friends and visitors, for short and long periods alike.

You have all played a valuable and important part in who I am today.

Love you,
Talor

CONTENTS

Introduction

Life can be meaningless if we live without stopping, without thinking, without feeling and without considering what we really want. I have discovered within me the power to bring meaning to life and become the person I want to be, using the tools of love, hope, faith and compassion.

The year 2008. The year when my life collapsed. I worked and occupied myself up to a point where I lost the distinction between the wheat and the chaff. I was a slave to my surroundings, my thoughts, my mind, my body and my soul. Out of disorientation, great pain, and the insights that came to my foggy mind while trying to escape from a trap whose name I did not know, and after having made radical and dramatic moves in my life, I was ensnared by a great despair which seized me with severe dizzy episodes that struck me and refused to leave.

Back then, I never imagined that, from my great desperation, a huge gift would pop out. I was hoping that something good would grow from this. Despite everything, I believed that if I fell into the abyss, I could only go up. How, when, and in what way, I did not know.

This is my life story, interwoven with questions and pondering, rattles and insights and shifts that were my part for many years, all the while not knowing what was wrong with me or why I was different from others. This is a true story, describing how I struggled, all my life, without success, to be like everyone else. How, for many years, my syndrome went undiagnosed, and how I experienced countless tests, diagnoses, treatments and mostly statements, such as, "Not much can be done... this is a part of life... it's all in your head... think positive... you have to learn to live with it," and so forth.

This is a story about a young girl, a teenager, a woman, a mother, an employee, who one day stood in front of the mirror and said, "No more!" I started a life's journey that was filled with uncertainty and ambiguity, and I did not know what was waiting at the end. My quality of life was poor. I felt like I was dying, but no! I wanted to live!

This is a story about me and the way I carried on, decisively and boldly, until

I found the proper solution, one that was good and right for me, for self-healing, happiness, joy and satisfaction and enjoyment of life, whilst fulfilling my dreams.

Success is measured in achieving the desired result. And there is no difference between failure and error. In neither case do we get the result that we want. Was I wrong? Did I fail somewhere along the way? For many years I thought I was cowardly, dependent, not good enough, not worthwhile, a person constantly in a "can't do" mode...

The difference is in the attitude, one person will tell himself: "I failed! I'm not good enough!" Another might say: "I was wrong. It hurts, but it's not too bad. I have learned and I'll keep going! Do I take a risk and try, even when the result is not guaranteed? Do I ask myself - what is the lesson I learned?"

I asked many questions when I felt I had failed and I did not get the result I wanted to. Was I wrong in my choices? Maybe so, but when I recognized the mistakes, I was ready to pay the price of uncertainty, coupled with determination and faith in achieving fulfillment in my life, as I felt I deserved, as I thought was right for me, as I wanted to feel. I was fighting for my life in a struggle that took its toll. I paid, and succeeded. I rehabilitated my health, my mind and my body. I have rehabilitated my life. In an amazing process, my life has been changed - my whole being was changed. If I could do it - anyone can!

One must find the strength that exists in himself. It does not mean it is a simple and easy thing. One must take a good look around, mostly within himself, and draw inspiration and strength.

My memory does not fail me. On the contrary, I remember every detail of my life, every event and experience which shaped my essence; days and nights, at home and at work, long walks and short through many events. Although the mechanism of repression that exists in humankind helps us to continue to deal with our daily tasks, it has not facilitated my function in the reality of life. Different experiences have influenced my life in a real, actual manner, and would not let me rest. I was a prisoner of my experiences, of my pains and thoughts, without any ability to repress them, address them, or bring them to account in the ongoing management of my life. I did not possess the powers or the tools I needed in order to deal with my troubles and make life easier, or to encourage myself to set out on a new, more optimistic, more joyous road - a road that would cause a dramatic change in my life. There was no one who would understand me and believe my troubles and feelings, no one who could see beyond my words and complaints, my cries and my pain. No one who'd say: "Wait a minute, maybe there's something else here... Let's take a deeper look. I believe you. Let's see what we can do together," or give support along the way - accompany, caress, wrap, comfort or love me, love me as I am - as a whole.

There was a huge void, disturbing, inexplicable, a great deal of confusion, ongoing frustration and especially terrible anger, a rage which bubbled and nibbled on every part of my soul and my body. Time and time again I was stunned when the floor dropped right from under my feet, the sky fell and... Start again..! What? How? Why? Where? What's happening to me? And why?

My strength was spent solely on proving to others, near and far, that I am normal. There are many like me. The attempt to resemble everyone else - friends, family members and others – charges a high price.

One day, after all, I decided to act. I decided to quit feeling sorry for myself and my condition; to start living as I deserved and could; to be happy; to cease being at war with myself and my disabilities. It was a battle of my strength versus my environment - with total helplessness crawling through my veins at every skirmish, though differing in intensity, and ruining everything good in me. I decided that if I was to fight, then I would do it for a better life, stocked with health, happiness, joy and satisfaction in every way and manner.

So I stood up on my feet and put it all behind me. The process has been long, hard, full of potholes, breaks and tears, and I did not know what was waiting for me at the end of the line or where the road would take me. But once I decided, I was determined to stay on the new path which I paved for myself, in which I feel free, creative and happy, reconciled with myself and my environment, at peace with the present, and able to make a difference and change in the lives of others.

The effort was worth it and it brought me to a place I never dreamed I would be in my life. That is why I wish to share my story with you, the readers, so that you will know the forces and capabilities that exist within us, that can help us to get out of any situation, and reach better and exciting districts of consciousness. There are few better examples than my own that express just how difficult and painful life can be. But I also know that you can do a lot in order to achieve change. If we only want to and decide upon it, we can change our thoughts and insights, we can change who we are. We will go through a process of change from thinking to self-talk, and then to action, for that is the determining factor. That is how we can live in a different, better reality, completely different from what we know.

I think my personal experience is what allows me to help others find the right tools for them, required just for them, in order to bring about their desired change, which they yearn for.

Memories of the Past

To be happy is an inner decision and every person, apparently, decides what level of happiness he is entitled to and deserves.

I grew up in a loving, warm house, born to Holocaust-surviving parents. My father and mother were born in the same small town in Poland and were friends when the war started. They had known each other since childhood. During the Holocaust, they hid in the ghetto for a long time and escaped together. They hid underground for eighteen months without fresh food or even a way to wash, and without adequate clothing for the harsh winters, like hunted animals. Both of their parents, along with my mother's sisters, were murdered before their eyes, and my parents had to flee from place to place in order to escape from the jaws of the murderous Nazis who threatened to exterminate all the Jews in Poland and other captured territories. My father, who was a resourceful man, finally managed to extricate himself, his sister and his girlfriend (that is, my mother) and was then drafted into the Red Army. In the meantime, my mother and my father's sister moved across Europe along with the refugees, and the thread between my parents was lost. At some point, my father defected from the Red Army in order to look for my mother, but there were no traces or clues or even a lead about her location. So my father travelled across the ruined nations of Europe, desperately trying to return to his lover and find out if she survived. Then suddenly, while staying by the Austrian border, he met a relative who told him that my mother was in Italy with his sister. My father was overwhelmed with joy and immediately began his journey to Italy. A few weeks later he located her and they fell into each other's arms. They got married immediately and, after a year, my only sister was born. Eighteen months later, they moved to Israel, where I was born six years after my sister.

All their lives my parents lived in Tel Aviv and never asked anything for themselves, only wanting to give me and my sister all kinds of advantages. When my father retired, he wrote the book "Between Hope and Despair", describing chilling stories about the Holocaust. Some of the stories were new to me and astonished me. Although they often talked with us about their lives at that time, only then did I realize that death had stared into my parent's eyes in every moment, through many long days, and how they lived with a sense of uncertainty and knew that they may not have much longer left to live.

All my life I've heard stories about the Holocaust, and they have influenced my life. How could they not? These were my dear parents, my immediate family, warm and loving. Every surviving acquaintance of my parents would often come to visit, and they were considered family. And what is it they would discuss? Their stories of survival, of course. Day and night we - my sister and I - were shrouded with accounts of dark horrors.

I remember nights in which I awoke, after having nightmares that made me sit bolt upright on my bed, shocked, and tried to go back to sleep, but it was impossible. In my dreams, I was persecuted by the Nazis. I hid from them. Sometimes I succeeded; often, I was shot. Again and again the dreams would recur at night.

I remember how, as early as in elementary school, I found it difficult to exercise. I felt pains in my body. The physical education teacher asked my mother to come to school to warn her that I was not participating in class as required. In fact, I simply could not perform the required tasks. It was hard for me to bend over, jump, and run… even my feet hurt. My eyes hurt. They burned and bothered me. I suffered from chemical allergies, hay fever and all kinds of other symptoms.

As a child, lots of little things bothered me and disrupted my daily life. I developed anxiety, distress and helplessness. I often did not understand what was happening to me. My mother took me to have tests, X-rays and physical therapy, and we visited various professional doctors.

Due to recurring pain and symptoms of panic that followed, my mother took me, when I was seventeen, to see a psychologist who treated me through a certain period of my life, following the recommendation of the school counselor. In her office, I remained silent at first, my mouth shut; no sound could get out of my throat for it was choked with tears of pain and frustration. My body was defying the questions of the psychologist who tried to smile and be cordial, to no avail. However, after a while I realized that if I did not talk and refused to release the secrets of my heart into the room, my condition would remain unchanged, and I would continue to suffer its various side effects. I began to cooperate, and she eased some of my constant distress.

I finished high school successfully. I was a student beloved by the teachers and I had many friends. I often wrote poetry and participated in school events. I was articulate in my writing and reading and I was socially dominant.

Like the rest of my friends, I joined the army. At the recruitment office, I asked to serve in the south because the doctors recommended that I should serve in the dry desert climate. Such a climate is healthier for those who suffer from hay fever. And so it was that I did my service in Sharm el-Sheikh at the southernmost point of our country. It was a beautiful place, with difficult field conditions and long shifts, and my profession required a high level of concentration. I suffered from eye strain and migraines that threatened to crack my head open, so I lived on painkillers because I tried to function and be like everyone else. On the outside I was cheerful and smiling, while on the inside, I cried, I suffered, and gritted my teeth.

I remember how frequently I visited the military clinic. There were days when I actually collapsed and I did not know if I could make it through the military service. The doctor had me do some tests, but they found nothing. And so I was taking painkillers to survive another day, another week, until I came home on weekends to Tel Aviv.

There were times I enjoyed the army - when I had moments of silence. I would sit in front of the sea, with a hat on my head and sunglasses on my nose because I could not stand the intensity of the sun, and relax. The sea, which was close to the base, was mesmerizing in its silence. I would watch the sun set, the mountains around and the breathtaking scenery of Sinai, and long for those moments when I could gather the mental strength to continue with military routine. I took a deep breath, unplugged myself for a moment from my obsessive thoughts and connected with the stunning view in front of me. I experienced moments of happiness and longing. I did a sort of meditation, alone, without knowing that was what I was doing, without noise or hustle, while briefly escaping the sensations of pain that bothered me most of the time.

The days passed, the pains came frequently, and I eventually asked to relocate to another base, more convenient and closer to my home in the center of the country. I realized that serving in the south did not resolve the symptoms from which I suffered. But at the new base, located more centrally, my eyes still burned and my head still ached. In the rooms where I worked, there were powerful neon lights that made my eyes hurt, poked at me and made me tear up. They made me dizzy. The long shifts and irregular working hours caused confusion in my body and hampered me physically. My pain was unbearable. I mostly kept to myself because I needed quiet. Despite all that, I survived my military service. I am adaptable by nature.

At the end of military service, I enrolled in a Bachelor's degree course at Ben-Gurion University in the Negev. Every Sunday, I took the train to Be'er-Sheva and went back on Thursdays to my parents' house. Along with my studies, I worked at three different jobs to support myself, coping with expenses such as housing, daily spending, leisure and more. Every day I was in constant motion and I would run here and there to fulfill all my tasks. I also went out for hikes with my classmates, but pretty soon I found that I was having a hard time keeping up… the intense heat in the south, the long, demanding hikes, and the equipment were too much for me. I gave up on visiting some of the attractions - travelling to them was just too complicated for me. I did not want to worsen my health, and I was afraid that I would be a burden on others.

The period of university education was so intense, I did not think about my condition all that much. I was very busy all week long, and obtained permission to work on Fridays in a respected institution; I needed to make a living, so I was a secretary for a day a week. My constant activity took a heavy toll, as I would take pills for the pain that would spread all over my body. I was sensitive to heat and cold, the muscles of my arms and legs ached, and I was dealing with the feelings in my body all the time. Wearing clothes irritated my body, while shirt labels scraped at my nerves. Shoes have always been a complicated matter. They were never comfortable - I had worn special insoles since childhood and it was hard to make my shoes go with the rest of my clothes. However, I did not give up on myself. I managed to gather up mental strength in order to receive my undergraduate degree successfully, and even added an additional year of education to achieve a teaching certificate.

After my undergraduate degree, I looked for a permanent job, and since I'd studied teaching, I received offers of teaching positions in some of the peripheral cities, such as Kiryat-gat and Ofakim. However, it was clear to me that I could not live far away from home due to the sensitivity of my condition, without even knowing, then, what it was. I lived with the feeling that I might be spoiled and delicate. To the various physical changes, a sore throat was now added. If I talked a lot during the course of a day, my throat would close up with pain. I suffered frequent infections in my throat and elsewhere in my body. I wondered how I could be a teacher and stand in front of a class for hours, when it was difficult for me to just to stand. I couldn't talk a lot... I lost count of the number of physical issues that I had to deal with.

I wanted to go back home, back to my parents' house. I was a home bird. I grew up as a princess and I was the spoiled little girl. Perhaps, I thought, I just wasn't designed to move away from where I grew up.

During my search for a job, I was told one day that there was a vacant position in the respected institution where I had worked as a student on Fridays, and the principal asked me to join the staff. When I told my parents, they strongly recommended that I accept. Working conditions there were very comfortable: favorable working hours, social benefits, air-conditioned offices, and more. It was more suited to my personality and my physical capabilities. I decided to accept the offer, and in order to take the role seriously and do it to the best of my ability, I immediately undertook some courses in this new field of work. After a further three years' study, I was fully qualified for my workplace and profession.

When I was very young I internalized an important piece of information that accompanied me throughout my life: if I sit back and wait for something to happen, it probably won't. I have to be the one to adjust my attitudes and actions for a better chance of a result.

Immediately after graduation, at the age of twenty-eight, I got married, a long time after my friends, many of whom had already had one or two children. It took time for me to graduate from my many years of study, to establish myself at work, and to meet my husband, whom I married in great love.

For ten whole years I was pregnant on and off. To this day, I do not understand where I found the strength because, physically, I was too weak. I know I had a strong desire to expand our little family. I had a strong desire to please my parents in any way possible and to atone for feelings of grief and sadness that had accompanied them throughout all their lives. I thought that every newborn child would make them happy and bring them joy.

Did that really happen? Was it sufficient reason? I don't know how to answer that in any other way, except to say that I felt a very strong need to give life again and again.

For most of my career, I worked almost full-time - thirty-four hours per week out of the more usual thirty-nine. This part-time position was made possible at my request and due to the fact that I was a mother with children to raise.

During my professional life I became dedicated to raising my children, and, thankfully, I was helped by a terrific nanny who pitched in to all of the household chores. Our hardworking nanny identified my difficulties, understood my needs and was attentive to my requests. She came to my aid in every possible way. She was an angel sent to me so that I could fulfill my duties as a mother and housewife well. Even today, we are strongly linked. Certainly, without her spontaneous help and vast kindness, I would have never succeeded in raising my children or functioning properly as was required of me in a respected institution. When I got back from work at noon, my four children would be taken care of. Some would be sleeping, having eaten and showered. This way, I could catch a half hour rest in bed. Without a noon nap, I cannot function properly in the afternoon and evening. I have to gather some strength and provide my body with much needed rest. About an hour's rest helps my body. I have had a nap at noon ever since I was a child.

Every now and then, when I held my children in my arms, I would remember the hard labor pains. Every time I was pregnant, there were many months during which it was considered to be a high-risk pregnancy. Following the birth of my first son, who was born quite low in weight, I needed my parents' help to recover. My mother supported me for several weeks and helped me take care of the new baby. My second pregnancy was disrupted by an infection in my body which harmed the fetus. The pregnancy ended in a miscarriage in the fifth month, and the frustration and sorrow were enormous. I wanted more children so badly.

A short time later I got pregnant again and, after nine months, my second son was born, also low in weight. And so, one after another, within very few years, my third and fourth sons were born after long periods of high-risk pregnancy, accompanied by close supervision and frequent examinations. The last pregnancy was cut short, and I gave birth to my fourth son prematurely; he was tiny and sweet and spent a few days in an incubator. Despite my physical exhaustion, I persisted bravely in all the births. True, I lay in bed, my swollen belly making day-to-day functioning difficult, and at times when the doctor allowed me, I even went to work. Yet it seemed as though the pregnancies were a kind of mental therapy, a kind of latent goal to expand our family and to bring joy to my parents. This would be a good place to mention that I was a sad girl - smiling, but sad. Ever since I can remember, I was looking for joy. These goals helped me cope with the physical tasks. Looking back, I do not know where I found the strength. Luckily, my personal doctor stayed by my bedside so I received treatment which suited my abilities and my low endurance.

I naively thought I could be in control of any situation, at any time, but I learned that it is one of the great illusions in life, and once in a while this illusion shatters. What then?

Eventually, I realized that nothing - no act, no effort - could really fill the vast space that had been created in the hearts of my parents, after all they had experienced in that terrible Holocaust. Much of their misery was passed on to me in the form of anxieties and fears . I accepted this as an integral part of my life and my heritage. I understood them and always felt great compassion in my heart for them. To my regret, I made them upset when my husband and I chose to separate.

We divorced after fourteen years when my eldest son was thirteen years old and my youngest boy was three. My physical and mental condition worsened and I realized that I had to re-establish my life quickly, in order to raise, care and educate my children.

I got myself together. After dividing our property, I bought a flat for myself and my children, an action that required a great deal of inner strength to withstand the heavy stress. In order to be able to stand the stressed period I became focused, and examined the way I would have to go in order to raise my children and allow them to live with a strong and functioning mother. At the end of it, the divorce eased my coping with life in general and the management of the house and raising children in particular. The constant pressure I had been under while married disappeared for a while; my husband lacked understanding of my hardship, my pain and my feelings, but I don't blame him, for he, like me, could not understand or know what was happening to me, as no one else around me could identify what was wrong with me.

The feeling that I did not like the way things were in my life, and knowing that I had the option to choose otherwise - since I am not an inanimate object incapable of acting - is what made me take a different path.

Shortly after our separation, I met my partner, who came into my life and the lives of my children, bringing great love. The days were filled with optimism and joy. I blossomed in the workplace, in my home and with my friends. This was a period of blossoming and hope for a better life. However, I still had to deal with my weaknesses and several intermittently appearing physical symptoms of sensitivity, and keep a daily routine while maintaining an intuitive balance, including a noon rest.

My children knew that I needed to rest at noon and cooperated with me, even though I had not spoken with them about my condition. I kept taking painkillers and functioned fully in every sense of the word. When the children grew older, they undertook various chores, such as taking out the garbage, filling the dishwasher, taking laundry from the dryer and organizing their rooms.

While working, raising and educating the children, and fostering a home and a romantic partnership, I continued to attend workshops and classes to relieve the various symptoms that would occasionally occur. I enrolled and participated in dozens of classes of various kinds of exercise, and gyms and private lessons, at huge expense. But I lacked perseverance. The pain prevented me from continuing to go to exercise classes, and from running, moving, stretching, bending, jumping around and coming home from class, happy and satisfied, like the rest of the participants.

After about ten happy years, during which our economic situation was better than ever, my relationship with my second partner ran aground. Later I could analyze what happened, but before I worked it out, I lived with many questions, wondering: What happened here? Unfortunately, I could not say and he - my partner in life - could not understand my condition, and I failed to explain to him what it was that I suffered from, exactly. Once, I even told him to stop asking me every day why I was crying. I cried because I was suffering and could not stand anymore, because the pain was destroying my life and gave me no peace, and I did not understand what was happening to me. Every day I woke up with something else hurting, and no one found out what was it that I had. Rather, the answer was that I did not have anything wrong with me. That was driving me crazy. I was helpless. I told him, "Don't ask me what's wrong and why I'm crying... I'm just hurting and I don't understand what's wrong with me!" Unfortunately, and to my dismay, he always claimed it was all in my head and that I should think positive and stop worrying, and not be so anxious. "Anyway," he argued, "you only die once." That was supposed to calm me down, but me - I wanted so badly to live. I knew that life is beautiful, and I felt I wanted to live it to the fullest, to do things, be someone, be happy, and I had children to raise and educate, and parents to whom I wanted to bring joy. I wanted everyone around me to be happy. Well, how could this be done? Would someone teach me how to deal with what was happening to me? How could I know?

For instance, whenever my partner wanted to go for walks, I found it difficult to join him gladly. I needed my siesta. And when I realized that an outing would deny me that rest, I would go into stress, anger and tense up - and the road from there to a fight was short. Another example - on Saturdays, when he woke up late in the morning after a week of work, and wanted to go for a walk or visit friends and enjoy the Saturday's rest, by this time I was already exhausted, having labored over household matters for the last few hours. Since I was a poor sleeper, I would wake up at dawn, tidying up the house as usual – this, after a night's sleep filled with awakenings, poor quality sleep, and often with terrible nightmares. Arguments would emerge between us because of his inability to understand why it was that I couldn't go for a walk, since I was already tired. Often, I had to stay at home, alone.

I suffered various phenomena all the time. Nevertheless, I would hang out with friends, but only up to the hours of noon, because I needed to rest. My partner, however, would only start his day when I was already tired and wanted to rest. He wanted to keep enjoying his day, and rightly so, and it took too much away from him to return home early in the afternoon. He also wanted to hike through winding trails on long walks, but that was not an option for me. I did not have the strength for all that walking around in the sun and certainly not for carrying my bag or going far. I had a hard time even standing, and when I did, even for a few moments, my feet hurt badly, and no one could understand that. Later in life, I read about the reason which caused this phenomenon and learned to deal with it. Until then, issues such as these created many conflicts between us.

There was a great love between us and I wished that we could have fun and, of course, that I could please him by participating in the things he liked to do. Also, I deeply wanted for him to be beside me, to support me, to love me as I am, and I didn't feel like it was so. I felt I needed to try and be someone else in order to feel worthy and successful, to feel like everyone else. And I tried to, and often I paid a heavy price in weakness and pain, sometimes many days later. Going out for entertainment tired me, but I could not stop. I later realized that it gave me strength, it was a kind of healing, a magic pill, a potion I longed to sip from more and more and never stop. Whenever I went out to a movie, a play or to relax at a coffee shop or meet friends, my mind was busy watching or talking, and somehow I had an hour of quiet and distraction from the pain. That's why I wanted it so badly. My body demanded it intuitively.

My frequent and lengthy use of painkillers caused side effects, and my body would go into a kind of vertigo, a vicious cycle impossible to get out of. In the aftermath of the storm, which came and went, I would go about my business diligently. I lived in a kind of denial. I didn't allow myself to be "sick" - it was out of the question. It seemed to me a terrible weakness and it really did not suit me. You could say that I ignored my body. The more my body screamed in pain, the more I ignored it and the more I grew angry with it for "bothering" me.

There were many days when I felt a kind of chronic flu coming and going. Every morning it raised its head and declared publicly: "I'm here and I'm not going to go away!" I had to visit the doctor alone. I did not want to involve those closest to me. I was rather embarrassed by the fact that I complained of pain all of the time. I didn't think that I needed any company or support since it was "my problem."

I functioned like a superwoman – one that could do anything! In the eyes of those around me, I was spoiled, a princess, a crybaby, a moaner and so forth. This increased my motivation to be the best at everything. Indeed, I was a sworn perfectionist and mostly hopelessly optimistic, because I always believed in my ability!

I cried a lot but kept on acting! I understand now, that was the wrong thing to do because it caused fluctuations and worsening of my condition. Every possible symptom appeared in my body: pain in various organs and each time in a different place, burning sensations in my muscles, various allergies, a burning sensation in my mouth, weakness, fatigue, anxiety, headaches, clumsiness, stiff and swollen fingers and a memory that began to fail me.

All that time, I searched for an answer as to my condition. I sought salvation. I attended many different workshops, read books and acquired an interest in alternative medicine. I went through various treatments in every field I came across along the way.

Later in life, I noticed a special phenomenon that repeated itself many times. I longed for organized trips abroad because I knew that the pains would disappear. Abroad, my body would be re-energized. I would wake up like everyone else in the early morning, get on the bus with the group and travel with them over many days. Come noon, of course, I would sleep for half an hour in the bus and gain new strength. I felt great. Abroad, nothing hurt me. But when I returned back home, my pains hit me again and reminded me that they were not going to disappear. They just took a vacation, along with me, abroad.

Later in life I realized that, overseas, I walked a lot, and that moving a lot was good for my body, although there were difficulties on a hard trip. I always found the things that I could do with everyone else. I gave up on some of the activities and so I'd sit and wait for the group in a café or at the hotel until they returned from the activities that were uncomfortable for me.

Health is necessarily influenced by the way we react to what happens in our bodies and its outward expression. If, day after day, I told myself the opposite of what I felt, if I kept doing things that did not suit me (although they were fine for everyone else) without realizing that it made my body a total mess, is there any wonder that I hurt to no avail?

I remember how, at my workplace, I was complimented on how well I looked, how well-groomed, how handsome and vital - but nobody knew how much I suffered. I kept my secret, never feeling the need to share my strain with my colleagues. More accurately, I was embarrassed. It was not seemly for my image or position. One day, after a lengthy deliberation with myself as my distress increased, I decided to tell my manager about my painful life. I went to his office, a little afraid, and asked him to listen to my needs. I asked him for help. I did not know what to do in order to continue working as is expected of someone in my profession. In response he promised, jokingly, of course, that he'd make sure to keep me as busy as possible, so that I'd forget my pains. This, indeed, was said jokingly, but who would have believed me anyway? I looked so good, and he, who knew me well, had seen how productive I was, and how diligent. Could he have believed that I had so much suffering, pain and sorrow in me?

The workload in my job was big, the responsibility was huge, my bosses trusted me, and I did not want to fail or disappoint them. I continued in my efforts to maintain my daily routine, went home in the evenings with my energy spent and with pains that stabbed my body, and I needed the pills to keep functioning. I did not want to disappoint the children or my partner, I wanted it to be "business as usual." I was always motivated to be the best in everything I did, but it came with a heavy price. I was sick for days. Sometimes the pills didn't help and I'd call a doctor to urgently come to my house and give me a pain relieving injection. Despite that, I tried not to miss any work days. I wasn't comfortable stating the reason for my absence every single time. I wasn't comfortable whining and complaining, knowing that people thought I was just a serial complainer with a screw loose…"Come on, crybaby… oh, sure… you look great, and you work like a bulldozer, so come on, enough with the stories…"□

The Diagnosis of Fibromyalgia

On one of my usual visits to the family doctor, once again struck by pain that went undetected by tests, he told me, "Well, as the tests didn't find anything, you probably have fibromyalgia."

I asked him, "What does that mean? What is it?"

And being a kind-hearted doctor, he explained that it's a kind of minor inflammation of the tendons and muscle fibers, and that there wasn't much could be done about it, and that I could read about it online if I wanted to know more.

An obvious conclusion is to start from the place you're at and use any means accessible, possible and practical in order to take the required action.

Of course, as soon as I got home, I went online to read about it. Muscle pain! Nice name. What is it? How do you treat it? What should I do next? From what I read, I found that it is not a disease, but rather a syndrome - a collection of varied effects. This syndrome is not dangerous, it is not malignant or, God forbid, fatal. That calmed me a little and I took the liberty of lowering a thin screen across my mind to close off the panic and fear that gripped me when I first heard the word 'fibromyalgia.'

I read a bit. I saw that most of my symptoms were mentioned there. I have fibromyalgia, what an honor! And? What do I do with it? Oh, that's an excellent question. There were several options, like going to a therapist, but I've already done that, I told myself. Maybe I'll go to hydrotherapy (exercising in hot water) - but I've tried that too. It's possible to take pills (antidepressants), but, I've already tried that and fortunately, only for a short time. I didn't respond to them well; they put me to sleep, so how was I supposed to get up for work? I couldn't take them and I stopped after the second pill. I understood the principle: numb the suffering person! That way, you don't feel the pain and everything is wonderful. What about Life? It goes on without you. Is this what I want? The question crossed my mind. No, of course not!

I left the whole story of this 'fibromyalgia.' What had it got to do with me? It did not relate to me, it was just a name and that was it. Doctors – though much appreciated - act according to what they know and understand: give a name to the problem, give out a pill. But I felt like it did not apply to me. I went on with my life as usual, but my mind already had a drawer called 'Fibromyalgia.' It was closed, and I never really thought about it too much. You could say I felt a kind of relief that I'd been diagnosed with something. But, still, it was all unfamiliar to me and I assumed a great sense of denial.

Obviously, I continued to visit the family doctor and again I underwent tests, X-rays, heart and lung ablation, and nothing was found. The doctor determined that I need to take pills for the pain. At first I did not understand what this syndrome is, and I gave no importance to it. It was useless to me. I visited websites and tried to extract information from various books, but did nothing with the information I gathered. My physical condition deteriorated, I cut back on my activities, and I felt exhausted. I wanted to work more, but my body was not listening to me. I was plunged into a daily battle for survival and my personal distress kept increasing. It was difficult for me to deal with the long hours at work. One day, I stumbled upon a notice inviting me to a workshop, to which I signed up intuitively, mostly because I had previously read two books related to it.

Breakthrough

My connection with imagination and reflection led to a spiritual and mental development, facilitated insights into my life, and granted strength to the will that was hidden inside me.

The year 2004 was the year in which a breakthrough in my life occurred. I participated in a workshop, one of many, called "The Artist's Way," an experiential workshop based on a book by Julia Cameron. The workshop was a path to independently rehabilitate the independent creativity latent in every human being, and the ideas it presented fascinated me. More than once I asked myself, Am I in the right place? I was employed by a respected institution - a bank - but does this kind of work suit me? Am I expressing my abilities?

The workshop encouraged participants to focus on different questions, and the most important was: are you satisfied with the long term results of your life? In short, are you satisfied with your life's progress - with where you are at this point in your life? Do you have any dreams? And what is your next dream?

Many questions popped in my head: What is 'your dream'? Who's dreaming? What about? What vision could there be in my life? I was busy all the time in the pursuit of healing and relief of my pain! What could I possibly dream about other than the possibility of getting up in the morning without any pain, and going through the rest of the day without fatigue and pain?

Once I asked these questions that popped up in my mind during the process of the workshop, I found no rest. The answers were written clearly, one by one, on the wall.

I was not satisfied. I had unexplained pains in different body parts, at different times. I visited too many doctors, spent too much time waiting for tests, wasted time on the phone waiting to make appointments with doctors and for treatment sessions, met with many therapists, spent a great deal of money on drugs, treatments and food supplements, and mostly wandered from workshop to workshop, one class to another, from the therapist to the analyst and from one alternative method to another combined with conventional medicine. My body went crazy. I didn't sleep at night. Most of the time I could achieve some relief, or at least some capability to tolerate the situation, but as for workable solutions – there were none. Those near and far to me did not understand me, did not attempt to take me seriously when I complained, or when I reacted with tears or sadness. My frustration was great; the pain had driven me insane and the whole situation was unbearable, bringing me to the brink of depression and despair.

No! No! I was not satisfied with the results of any actions I had taken. That thought would not let go. Despite the many actions I took on all levels - the results were not satisfactory.

There seemed to be something else that was outside the scope of my experience and that I had yet to solve, and that was why my life was the way it was, a lasting physical and psychological suffering with signs of desperation. And hope… none.

Of course, the questions in my head all along were: What else should I do? Why have I failed to learn? What haven't I learned? What is hidden to my eyes? Who is the one I have yet to find? (A therapist? A wizard?) Whose hands hold the solution? How naive my thoughts were.

I suddenly realized that I had never taken the course of action that was right for me, due to my own false thoughts about myself, due to the false thought of others about me and from a basic misunderstanding of the needs of my body and mind. My naive way of thinking was that something external to me, some external entity, would 'take it' from me; I believed that 'others can help me more then myself' (doctors, therapists, pills, supplements, etc.) without me changing anything about my way of thinking, without doing something other than I'd already done. My will was to stick to what was familiar, walk the same way , 'like everyone else' and not to appear abnormal. This was driven, of course, by a complete lack of faith in myself and my abilities. All of these naive thoughts had brought me this far and I was not happy with the results…

I suddenly realized that I did not like what was happening in my life, and I must find the strength to change my actions. Otherwise, I'd get the same result over and over.

It was clear to me that I would not give up, but there was no way I was going to go on like this! But what would I do instead? My head was preoccupied with these thoughts while I got involved with my individual process in the workshop and performed my homework as required. With every meeting, I dove deeper into the fiber of my soul and confronted my doubts.

And then a great enlightenment occurred in me. I got it. I arrived at a very important insight that changed the course of my life, formed a clear turn in the path I was to take, leaving my past behind at some point, while the present had become full of contentment, and the future brighter than ever, with the possibility of flourishing! Hope seemed very worthwhile and a light shimmered at the end of the tunnel.

The Birth of the Transformation

My knowledge was not achieved by chance alone. I sought it passionately and diligently since I was a girl, and as I got older, I persevered even more to acquire knowledge relevant to my life.

I clearly knew that my poor health was preventing me from living happily, and that my environment was influenced by how I felt and, certainly, I could go no further in that direction. It was clear that the path on which I walked had to change direction, but what should I do? I'd already seen so many experts, experienced a range of treatments and tried different methods. It was still there! And I did not even know what 'it' was. Seem complicated? I felt so too. I did not know what I was facing. Nonetheless, I made a decision.

I decided to focus on my health. I decided I had to improve my health, come to grips with what was wrong with me, what it was that was running my life and find out whether or not I even had some recognized condition. How could I get out of the intolerable situation I was in? This situation had lasted for a long time. Back then, I did not know that the phenomenon from which I suffered had plagued me since childhood. At that at point, I thought that I'd begun to suffer only recently. I was, really, only concerned about the period during which my condition worsened, when it became harder to tolerate than before. I realized that until I was healthy, I could not continue to do the daily chores, or be the sort of woman I wanted to be: happy, optimistic, creative and happy, capable of contributing to society.

I decided that I was the one who should take different action than I had before, if I wanted to get results different from those I had got thus far...

The decision, however, was just the beginning. I did not know that by actually making the decision, I had jumped into a raging river that would take me to places that I never dreamed of at the time when I decided. Glad that happened!

Later on, we were hit very hard. In 2005, it became clear that my partner had a terrible disease. It also became clear that the signs of his disease had started a few years earlier, but that he had not related them to any disease. The difficulties he experienced in everyday functioning were added to my own. This blow severely affected my health, but I continued to be act as if I was Superwoman. His illness won't change the integrity of our family, I thought. We'd continue to function and make every effort to treat him and live like an ordinary family. His ongoing refusal to accept the disease and the treatment - more precisely, his denial of the symptoms of the disease and its effects on us as a family – threatened our good relationship, which started going downhill despite the great love between us.

The tragedy was at full strength. The house was filled with a difficult atmosphere, and I still needed to take care of my children, manage the household and go to work as usual, and was concurrently worried about my elderly parents, to whom I devoted special time every week, though I never gave up visiting and calling them. I persevered with my strong desire to please them in every way I could. I hid my partner's serious illness from them, because I did not want to upset them and did not want them worrying about me. This was difficult - almost unbearable. Over time, they noticed problems happening, and they started asking me questions about him, but I denied there was any problem and avoided providing answers. It was important to me that their last days be as relaxed and happy as possible. They grew older and needed care too – I helped them get to the doctor's, paid them frequent visits and gave them general assistance.

Experimenting is a challenging and unrelenting experience, because, at first, there is innocent or deliberate action and then an examination of the things that are happening - lack of faith, fears - and in the end, you learn a lesson.

Meeting up with a friend, who was also an alternative therapist, led to a conversation in which the word fibromyalgia came up. This friend pointed out to me that there was a clinic at Ichilov Hospital run by a specialist in fibromyalgia, and she recommended that I make an appointment to see if, in fact, that was what I was suffering from. Was this coincidence, or was it an opportunity?

After seeing so many different doctors and suffering so many disappointments and much frustration, I decided that I had nothing to lose. What's the worst that could happen? Another visit to a doctor - and maybe this time something would turn up and open my eyes? I decided I should check to see if I really was a victim of this syndrome, as suggested by my doctor recently.

Although my friend warned me that the waiting time for a diagnostic appointment was lengthy, within three weeks I was at the Rheumatology Clinic at Ichilov Hospital. I was examined by a fibromyalgia specialist, who patiently listened to me for a long time. I described my story over the years and the various phenomena that bothered me. I'd brought many documents with me - results of tests and summaries from doctors - but he used a small device to press eighteen different points on my body. Every time, it hurt me very much. It was surprising, because the pressure wasn't great; my sensitivity was probably very high.

At the end of the examination, the doctor determined that I definitely suffered from fibromyalgia: pain in muscles and fibrous tissues. He briefly explained the meaning of the illness and its consequences, and gave me a letter confirming that I have the syndrome (it was like receiving a diploma at the end of a college course). In the letter, there were recommendations for seeing a psychologist (I had done this already, remember?), a referral for hydrotherapy treatment (does this sound familiar?) and a recommendation to take medication (Eltrolit), for pain relief. In case none of the above helped, he recommended that I take a stronger medication called Cymbalta.

Courage! As I overcame fear to achieve something important to me, did that mean I am a brave person?
Most of the time I thought I was a coward trying to hide an unexplained defect that exists in me.

To tell the truth, when I left the clinic, which I had attended alone, without the support of any member of my family (for I hadn't told them I was going to see yet another doctor) I suddenly felt very relieved. I was immensely relieved, as if a heavy stone had been lifted from around my neck, as though the heavy, gray cloud that had shrouded me for months and years was dissolved away in a second.

All of a sudden, there was a name to all these bizarre phenomena that I experienced. Suddenly, I wasn't 'abnormal'; suddenly it was not 'all in my head'; suddenly, I was just an ordinary woman who had fibromyalgia syndrome. And as I understood from the kindly doctor, I suffered from a syndrome, meaning a collection of symptoms, and not a disease, and it was not malignant, not terminal, not dangerous - but very disturbing and troublesome, and it affected my quality of life. Finally, there was a definition to all of the phenomena and symptoms, aches and pains.

There is no doubt that in every moment today, we are flooded with enormous amounts of information that sometimes can make us think we are losing our common sense.
Focused information may result in clarity of thought and aid concentration toward our goal.

Where am I headed?? Now what do I do?

It was only many months later that I learned that all of the medical examinations and all of the symptoms and the phenomena yet to be described here had a certain reason or cause behind them.

I got home, told my spouse what the doctor had said and sat down to go online and read what was written about it. I wanted to understand exactly what the doctor meant. There were articles on the subject. Some were confusing, the contents vague, and most talked about specific symptoms and focused on the muscle pain. But there were also other similar phenomena mentioned, all of which I had experienced. Also, there were all kinds of suggestions for treatments to relieve the sensations and pain, but I'd tried most of them. I somehow let the days go by, and didn't think too much about it.

This time, once again, I failed to understand what this syndrome was, and I didn't attach much importance to it. But I had the diagnosis written in black and white, and I could no longer ignore it completely, yet still it was useless to me. I know myself: if I'm hurting, I take a pill and move on full steam ahead. It hurts again, so go visit the doctor again... tests, X-Rays, pills, time off work, and all over again. What had changed? Well, I got a name for all of the pain. And pills. So..?

I went back to browsing websites, trying to extract information from various books, but did nothing with the information I gathered. My physical condition deteriorated, I cut back on my activity, and I felt exhausted. I wanted to do more, but my body was not listening to me. I was fighting a battle for daily survival and my distress was escalating.

Meanwhile, I kept going to the workshop "The way of the artist" and the more time passed, the more I was committed to it. And since I'd already made a preliminary decision to focus on my health, and since I was determined to take care of my health and promote it to a state which would allow me to function like all other people, and now I had committed to my decision to get better - I took half an Eltrolit pill as the doctor had prescribed.

That night I slept well. Yes, I slept really well, but when morning came - a time when I normally jumped out of bed seconds before the alarm went off, time when I started to run around the house to get four children to school with their sandwiches, and having drunk, eaten, made beds and got the dryer going, leaving the house shining and ready for when we returned to it at noon to continue our busy, daily routine - that morning, I could not jump! I was sleepy and fuzzy and all I wanted was to be left alone.

I am a very responsible woman. I got up all blurry, performed my duties as usual and I got to work somehow. Half a day passed with difficulty in coping with the unrelenting blur that seized me. I thought to myself that it was just a matter of a day or two, I'd get used to the drug and everything would change for the better.

The next day, the same situation occurred. I felt terrible arriving at work in that condition and having to explain to my boss about my situation, and having to ask for special consideration.

That evening I made a decision. No! It's not for me! I am not ready to be drugged on the altar of my health. This was not what I wished for. I wanted to be healthy, and not suffer any more pain. Nor was I willing to be drowsy, sleepy and half stoned! This did not seem to be the way to go.

I immediately stopped taking the pills and I knew in my heart that I would never again consume pills that had harmful effects on me or might cause side effects. It was clear that this was not the right direction for me.

The days went by. One day I heard about a fibromyalgia syndrome support group held in Ichilov Hospital. A notice jumped out at me from one of the websites.

A "coincidence" do you think? We'll see just how many more times coincidence played its part and led me to where I am now.

An ancient Chinese proverb says that in order to move a mountain we have to start with the smallest stones.

I called to find out what I could about it. I spoke with a cheerful woman who led the workshop, who assured me that I could recover from fibromyalgia, and the proof was that she no longer suffered from it, so she was running this support group at Ichilov Hospital.

I never hesitate. I know an opportunity when I see one. When it is clear to me that the right thing present itself. A kind of intuition or optimism, related to an old faith of mine, sustained a feeling that there was someone who always watched over me from above. If this workshop had crossed my path, I'd be there.

How am I going to manage this? The workshop lasted three months, once a week, three hours in the afternoon. I work and when I come back, I have to rest because I'm tired... and the children... the house... and the chores? And I have to drive to the center of Tel Aviv and find parking. How do I do it? The task seemed very difficult, virtually impossible to me. Herzliya to Tel Aviv during the rush hour? I'd have to leave very early to get there by five o'clock. A sense of helplessness and despair swamped me at the very first instant.

Still, I did not give up and I went to the workshop once a week for three whole months. And slowly, it hit me very strongly. It penetrated my head and created an opening for a new path. Till then, I'd drifted through life with thoughts on how to get well, stop these pains and live normally that were hardly groundbreaking.

While having support conversations with the other women in the room, all of whom were in one state of misery or another - suffering, hurting, with nobody to understand them - I felt like there was one language understandable to all; there was love and encouragement and a great understanding that I was not alone, that there were other women like me, suffering from the same differing and bizarre symptoms. They came from all over the country and were of different ages, and all sang the same chorus: want to but cannot. The physical, mental and emotional difficulties, the frequent pain, the plaguing symptoms and the lack of knowledge and understanding of those around us were enough to cause insanity, and despair was dangerously close.

Lizzie, our amazing instructor, gently and quietly, calmly and professionally, led us from one meeting to another with confidence and she propped us all up with her listening ear and endless support during the meetings and afterward.

Towards the end of the workshop, a joint meeting was held with all the girls in the group, and each was asked to bring a family member or two, from those closest to her. The professor, who was an expert on the syndrome, gave a formal lecture in which he explained to the audience what fibromyalgia is, what causes it, how important the help and support of family and relatives is, and how you should behave with patients around the house and outdoors. I brought my partner and my eldest son, who was twenty two.

I do not know what impression the words of the professor left on them. Initially, I felt a bit more empathy and goodwill from them, but the daily routine did not leave a large margin of compassion from my family circle. Even though I explained to my children what I had been diagnosed with, I felt no drastic change in our relationships, and received no more special help than before.

One day I realized that in order to come out of the difficult situation my body had gotten into (My body. Not me! I was the cute girl, a mother, a wife, my parent's daughter – I was myself! My body was the problem), I needed to reduce stress and tension significantly. I should take extreme action, have a life makeover, and bring about a big change to bring the desired results - meaning recovery!

Doubts and Fears

I was attacked by hard feelings and by the clear knowledge that there might be risks along the way that, maybe, I couldn't afford to take. On the other hand, there were certainly other risks that I couldn't afford NOT to take and that was the case. It was now or never!

I had been working at the bank for thirty years. I'd finished my bachelor's degree with a fourth year teaching diploma, and I'd also studied for three further years and achieved a banking diploma. I also participated in different courses and a number of workshops. I was in a senior position in the branch's service department, along with my duties as secretary and office manager for the branch manager. I was a valued employee, popular, industrious and creative. I demonstrated initiative and I had many more years ahead of me before I retired.

A hard and unacceptable thought began to run through my mind. Pros and cons… could I retire? What would I do with my life? I had a good salary, there were social benefits, a social life and business trips abroad. I had a diverse role, and I did like getting up in the morning for work. I loved what I did. Just like that - up and leave? Walk out? I'd heard that some women from the support workshop were already in the process of early retirement and some workplaces already recognized the syndrome as a valid cause.

I immediately removed the thought from my head. No! I'm not taking that route. Wait a minute - maybe I should check out the idea? My mind was full of thoughts regarding the choices in front of me. Who would listen to me anyway?

I could identify with the fact that most people experience change as a threat rather than a challenge. In a situation where fears of abandoning that which is familiar and comfortable arise, it was hard to see change as an opening for the creation of something new and exciting.

I was finding it hard to cope with the long hours and I felt my strength running out. Every day, it was harder and harder to get out of bed, and it was unbearable trying to make it through to the end of the working day. By afternoon, I was already exhausted and the pain was melting the cells of my brain. I dropped files and folders, I felt my memory fail me often and I lost confidence in myself. My suffering was excruciating.

Whenever I was at work I wanted to go home, but at home I just walked around in pain, sadness and anger. The quantity of anger bubbling in me cannot be described. I was upset at myself that I couldn't do what I wanted to, I was angry at everyone around me for not understanding what I was going through, and I was angry at my spouse for not being there for me in the past and certainly not now, when he was dealing with his own illness and was in need of my support himself. Every little noise threw me off balance, and there were noises aplenty: the gardener mowing the lawn or using his blower; garbage men collecting trash and emptying it into the truck, then reversing down the street with loud and piercing beeping; the neighbor's dog barking all the time... My nerves were on edge most of the time, and I was a painful bundle of damaged nerves, unraveled and crying.

That's when I decided to check my options to reduce the stress and the tension that were an integral part of my life, as I knew I must if I want to be healed.

I had to go to an occupational therapist. I made an appointment and brought with me all my documents: X-rays, observations, and summaries of the syndrome. The doctor asked me several questions, and I described my condition. He didn't look at the documents I brought. He did not need convincing - he saw and heard me. For most of the conversation, I cried. I almost could not speak. I told him how much I loved my work and how I felt like my body was betraying me and how frustrated I was by the gap between my desires and capabilities.

The doctor announced immediately that I needed to reduce my working hours. How do I do this? I am the boss's secretary! If I'm not around when he needs me, what does he need me for at all? I could not agree to the doctor's proposal to stop working, split my hours or significantly reduce the amount of hours at work. No! No! That's out of the question!

Eventually, I accepted a doctor's note that officially recognized that I should work one hour less a day. I thought to myself: I'll divide my free time, and work half an hour less at noon, and I'll get another half hour later in the afternoon. This would allow me greater scope to relax in the afternoons at home and reduce my stress.

The next day I went to see my boss. I hesitantly stuttered that I had permission to work an hour less. He didn't say much, and I slipped out of his room and decided that I might have permission, but I'd try not to use it. I did not feel comfortable to use the permission.

Any change requires absolute attunement and certainty that change is possible. But me? I was afraid of my own shadow!

At first I did not take advantage of the doctor's recommendation because I felt uncomfortable about it in front of my boss and colleagues, but as the days became more difficult and I saw my body starting to collapse from overload, I had no choice. One day, I decided to use the certificate and told the boss I would henceforth start to work one hour less each day.

And so, for six months, I worked one hour less a day, on the recommendation of the doctor, and then the certificate was extended for another six months.

Every day I would go home earlier than usual, trying to ignore the looks of my colleagues. I felt enormous shame and lack of support; certainly, no one could understand why the boss's secretary was allowed to go home early, and come in later than everyone else. The whispering behind my back and the looks I drew caused terrible stress. There was huge pressure from all directions. On the one hand, I left earlier to go home, but on the other, I wanted - and, of course, felt obliged – to finish all my daily work in less time every day. How could this situation reduce stress? On the contrary, I tried even harder to perform my responsibilities well, to prove that I needed less time to do it all and then more. Ha ha! Heaven laughed. The symptoms intensified, I was on the verge of collapse and, back at home, things were difficult.

The certificate I received from the occupational therapist was valid for several months, at the end of which I went back to see him. He spoke to my heart and advised me to stop working. "Split hour working is not suitable for you," he said. "Continuing to work will make it difficult for you to cope with the syndrome. You must change your way of life."

I was shocked. Stop working at the age of fifty-five? What would I do at home? I sat there weeping in his room, frantic with grief, alone, without a kindred spirit to consult with. When I calmed down, I thought a little and asked him to compromise, to certificate me to work just five hours a day. I was not ready for early retirement. I was afraid that at home, I would become introspective, and in general I'm a person who likes to work and learn. Why would I stay at home?

I submitted the certificate, and undertook to work only five hours a day. Yes, I gave up. I chose not to see and hear what people said, or what they thought of me. This was how it was to be and I had to learn to adapt to it. That's what I thought to myself.

And indeed, for a while I felt relief from my pain. My condition improved; I tried to do some sports-walking, and I didn't stint in my devotion to work – I still gave it my all, showing that I was trying hard and wanted to be successful despite my condition. Indeed, I was managing well, even when under pressure, though I sometimes forgot things and occasionally dropped heavy binders. My frustration stemmed from the gap between what I wanted to do and what I could do. Everything I did came with great agony.

In addition to all the symptoms and my sensitivity, during the last twenty years I'd occasionally had lesions caused by sun damage removed from my nose and face. Sun damage???

I regularly argued with my dermatologist and plastic surgeon. They insisted these lesions were caused by exposure to the sun in childhood and adolescence. I told them it couldn't be. From an early age, I remembered wearing a hat and sunglasses on my head. My skin could not bear the heat of the sun and my eyes were sensitive to light. I'd had to hide, so I couldn't tan in the sun like the rest of my friends. Yet, due to my high sensitivity, lesions would emerge, occasionally needing to be removed. Every time I underwent invasive treatment, I was signed off work to recover. However, I did not use all of those sick days; I always went back to work earlier than expected.

It turns out that one can learn anything in order to achieve a goal. I wanted to be healed and have the pain and fatigue stop, and I wanted to find joy.

Over the years, I studied different healing methods. I wanted to be able to take care of myself as necessary, and so I learned Reiki, Theta Healing and Bio-ergonomics, energetic methods which I used to help myself and my family. I also learned to use different types of awareness cards and utilize messages. I took interest in the different theories and I often read about Zen Buddhism, Ayurveda, Chinese medicine, diet by blood type, and more. I experienced different types of alternative medicine, I studied body language and was interested in Neuro-linguistic programming (NLP).

Furthermore, I read about holistic pulsing and underwent treatments that didn't necessarily support my situation, and sometimes even worsened it. I tried acupuncture, but I did not like the pricks of the needles. They hurt a lot. I was interested in the reasons for high cholesterol and the possibility of decreasing it, and I read books and articles about the body's organs and their function. I read about various medications and their side effects, and I was interested in the various types of alternative healing.

In 2007 a routine checkup at the dermatologist's revealed that I need urgent surgery, due to a local lesion on my nose which was suspected to be dangerous. I walked around angry and frustrated. I have to go through all this now? Another surgery? I'd already said I'd had enough. This had to stop! Why was I going through this again?

I didn't tell a soul, except for my sister, who accompanied me into the operating room. The doctor thought it was something really small, but to our horror, the surgery went on and on and eventually I had to get a skin graft from my ear to my nose. It was a nightmare. I was scared, sad, and I was terrified about how I would look. My spouse, who was at work during the operation, looked for me at home and found out I was in the hospital. He arrived scared and shaken. Why hadn't I told him? But I didn't want to share this with anyone:

What, again I'm the nuisance? Yet again, I have to go into hospital? Once again, I'm to be pitied? I preferred to go only with my sister, finish it quickly and go home quietly. But this time? This time it was a very big deal.

At home, on my pillow, when I arrived home, exhausted after long hours of surgery with bandages over most of my face and ears, I found a most exciting letter from my youngest son, who was fifteen years old and a high school student. This was a letter of love and appreciation to me - a heartbreaking letter. My heart trembled with joy and happiness at all reinforcing words that were written there, and my eyes watered with large, hot, salty tears, yet I could not move a muscle in my face due to the stitches, and had to restrain myself from crying terribly. Yes, my son had also been upset at not knowing where I was, and when he realized I had undergone surgery and I was about to come back home, he wanted to please me and wrote these warm and loving words. This was his way of telling me that he understood, even if I kept it all to myself. This letter brought lots of light into my life, as well as the hope and knowledge that I could not stop along the way and that I needed to fully recover. There was someone waiting for me, who needed me, who loved me.

Once again I returned to work earlier than the doctor ordered. I walked around with dressings on my face for a few weeks until I recovered. The scar remained red for a long time. But the scar on my face was nothing compared to the scar etched on my heart. Following this surgery, my heart did not stop bleeding. I did not understand what was happening or why... I'd been through every possible treatment. I'd reduced my working hours. I'd attended a meditation class for several years to relax my body; I was becoming more aware, I read books. So what was wrong? What hadn't I done yet?

The relationship between my partner and me continued to deteriorate dramatically. We lived out an impossible scenario that affected us adversely and, although we loved each other, we could not bridge the gulf between us due to the lethal combination of his serious and escalating illness and my fibromyalgia symptoms. My anger skyrocketed. I could not live any more in my own skin, while hot flashes started to strike me and my body flamed and burned. My mouth ached and my palate burned me constantly. I saw many doctors and I even went to the oral and maxillofacial faculty at Tel Aviv University for examination. Everyone unanimously declared these symptoms as characteristic of the syndrome and stated there was nothing they could do. I consumed food supplements and herbal remedies, I took various foods off my diet and added others to which I was not accustomed, drank silver water, and avoided unhealthy foods, but nothing helped. Sometimes, I would feel a temporary relief from the symptoms, but most of the time, they just got worse.

I suddenly noticed that my memory was growing weak. I was so scared that I made an appointment at Beilinson Hospital's Memory Clinic. I thought I had Alzheimer's. I made my way there with great difficulty, imagining what my life would be like if I was, indeed, struck by this disease. But the doctor who examined me stated that there was nothing wrong with me, apart from a high level of stress. "The moment you reduce the stress, your memory will return to you. Reduce your stress levels. I'll see you in a year," she said with a sympathetic smile. I calmed down. Sipping a glass of water and left on my own, I realized once again, for the umpteenth time, that I finally needed to act to significantly reduce the stress in my life.

British psychologist Anna Freud said, "I used to seek power and security outside of myself, but they are inside. They had always been there."

I did not have the strength to continue my difficult life. I was confused and I wanted a change. I cried for many a night, tears pouring down my face. My pillow knew many secrets and soaked up many tears. I buried my head in it, to forget the world around me, to forget the situation, and imagine my face as it was not so long ago. I wanted to turn away from the reality of life. I wanted to remember the distant past. Now, every day was too much to bear, as was every hour and every moment. Thoughts raced through my mind without letting go. What am I to do? What more can I do to in order to get peace and quiet?

At that time, my beloved mother was rushed to the hospital and it turned out that she had to undergo open-heart valve replacement. The whole family rallied, and the tension was terrible. We were very scared. She was eighty-seven. We sat with her constantly, in shifts. My father, who had been blind for several years now, remained at home with his devoted caregiver, and so we skipped between the hospital and my father's house. Those were stressful days, fraught with concern. They exacerbated my condition which was shaky even before this most recent drama, following my last surgery from which I had not yet recovered.

There was the time I walked around the hospital and saw many patients confined to their beds and thought about my life, about my sensations, about my suffering and everything I was going through, and I remembered that I'd promised myself I would focus on my own health. I remembered I wanted to do everything I could to get well. And what else had I not yet done? The question kept going through my mind, and the answer was quick to follow. When it arrived, I did not hesitate for long. This was the most significant decision in my life. Once I chose this option, I clung to it however I could, in every moment, and never let it go. There were ups and downs, but I stuck by my new path.

The Transformation

Where would I get to? I did not know. However, it was clear that those who are sufficiently determined will reach their destination, and I was already determined.

I had decided to step down from my job at the bank and leave in order to take care of myself, encouraged by the stories I'd read or seen on TV about people in Israel and abroad, people who were in difficult situations and had made a decision and had stuck to it until they brought about the success they had sought. I decided that I, too, could succeed.

One by one, I picked up all of the documents I had, all of the evidence of my suffering over the years and I got myself once more, as faded as an autumn leaf, to the occupational therapist.

In just a few minutes, I had in my hands a letter containing the unequivocal diagnosis: an immediate loss of ability to work. At that time, I did not understand the full impact of this diagnosis. The doctor asked for the fax number of the bank and sent the manager the letter I had just received. He wished me luck, asked me to take care of myself and advised me to conserve my energy and take care of my health.

The next morning I went to work as usual. An hour later, I was told over the phone that I had to leave the branch and that in a few hours a letter signed by a doctor would arrive at the bank confirming the validity of the occupational therapist's letter as stated: an immediate loss of ability to work. This was immediate, meaning I was no longer able to work and should go home. Just like that, after thirty years of work, at the age of fifty-five, and with many years still ahead of me, I had to retire unexpectedly.

What thoughts went through my mind in those moments? I don't remember much except for the fact that I wanted peace and rest for my painful spirit. Nothing else mattered to me. These were rare moments of shock, relief, release and emptiness all mixed together. I wanted to finally take care of myself, of my pain. This was an opportunity to focus on myself. My children were all grown and I could make time for myself, and if I was not working, I could devote this time to healing.

How? This I did not yet know, but I felt a huge relief. I felt free. I had no duties requiring me to get up in the morning and start running! How would that look? How would it feel?

For the following few mornings, I continued to wake up early - I'm a woman of action. However, the very fact that I was free and I did not have to start running, get things done, get to work on time, be responsible and attentive, or provide for the needs of others such as work colleagues, brought with it great spiritual gain and an actual relief.

I often asked myself: am I endowed with what it takes in order to become successful? This is an important question one should ask, and as I recall, the response to my thought was positive.

I read many inspiring stories that fuelled my determination to succeed. I connected with books that spoke to my heart, reassured me and gave me hope. I settled into a state of temporary uncertainty, and I believed in my ability to succeed. If others can, so can I. I repeated and memorized this to myself. I knew I was embarking on a new road, filled with uncertainty and embodying many opportunities for change in my life.

The next morning was painted with cautious optimism. I knew that I would never have to go to work again. My head wasn't as busy with thoughts. I recalled how at eleven o'clock in the morning, at work, I would feel a weakness all over my body and want to go home; I remembered how I realized, after visiting doctors, that my immune system was weak and my mental state wasn't good. I did appreciate my workplace for providing me with appropriate conditions, but my forces were spent. I hoped to have better days ahead of me. But how would they will be better? This, I did not know. It was clear to me that in order for them to be better, I would have to do something. But what? What should I do?

I took responsibility for change, for it was clear to me that the nub of the matter was not what happened to me, but what I did with it, and I already understood that I'd acquired a lot of information and now I must take responsibility for creating the change I so longed for!

A few days later - which were not without pain - and with my mood swinging between happiness at being free from the routine of work and suddenly having no fulfilling activity, I made an appointment with the psychologist who had treated me on and off for many years. I'd read all of his books over the years and I knew his views regarding changes in peoples lives. His fascinating book "A Friendly Change" reflected the changes in my life. I liked his approach, since it was very friendly and unconventional. Yes, for many years I would consult with him, consolidate and clarify important issues, gain encouragement and learn in order to improve my abilities and achieve something I did not yet know what it would be. I was left, after thirty years of intensive work, with a huge void, with recreational time I had no idea how to fill, except for the pain that would not go away and housework, as well as taking care of my children who still lived at home, and the constant care of my aging parents. My first discussion with him left me stunned and in awe. I shared with him my plight, along with my great happiness at being retired - and he?

He actually painted a dark image in my imagination of a future reality in which I would need to deal with the syndrome and the inaction. "Retirement may be harmful for you," he said. "You might spend your life visiting doctors and therapists, and with time on your hands, your pain may claim your attention and occupy and consume your time. You'll have to fight your pain more. Take care of your children, your parents and your partner. You'll spend a lot more time at the HMO and it will be your main occupation, unless..."

This time, I left his office in a very emotional state. I went in strong and came out weak. My hurting soul only asked for peace and quiet, but it was storming. My blood pressure rose, and like a sleepwalker in a frenzy, I went up the steps to the parking lot adjacent to the building, quickly got into my car and drove off.

I turned on the radio and listened to the music. Luckily, I have faith in myself and my abilities, despite the symptoms from which I suffered. I have always tried to prove to myself that I can overcome anything, and so it was in this case - I wanted to show my psychotherapist that he was wrong. I thought to myself: what do I want to do with my life? The children were grown already, I had a steady income, and I was free to choose.

I'll show him… What he predicted won't happen to me… I'm not like that… I'm hardworking, punctual, and I love working. Why would I ever spend time at the HMO? No way is that happening!

Another important decision of mine: the only person whose opinion really should have any effect on my life was me. I would make my own decisions and I would put them into action and it would not matter to me what someone else had to say about me or thought of me.

The psychologist did paint a black picture, but I decided it would be painted in happy, cheerful colors. He was the angel sent to me from Heaven. His was the voice in the wilderness that warned me that if I continued on with life as before, I'd collapse someday, especially after I retired. I could identify where there was a distortion between what he claimed might happen to me and my certainty that my life was going to be full of contentment, joy and vividness. I'd told him about fibromyalgia and explained the diagnosis and symptoms. He knew me of old and was aware of "my stories," as he called them, but I had a feeling he did not really believe me. Yet I was drawn to meet him because I felt there were things he said that spoke to my heart, that were true for me. Call it intuition, call it guidance from above. I knew inside me that his words were directed to me and to a certain extent, it was my choice. Accordingly, I kept going to meetings and doing my homework, according to his methodology. They were only a few sessions, about which you will read later on, but they made a long term impact.

On one occasion, during a conversation, the psychologist, my dear and brave friend, said something that firmly determined my future path: "I don't understand the syndrome, and I'm not even sure it's something real. I read about it and I was interested to understand what it is. From what I can make out, I'm telling you that you alone can heal yourself. You alone know how you feel, only you know for sure what's right for you and what's not, and therefore you are the one who can make things happen. In other words, heal yourself!"

American philosopher Jim Rohn said that ideas are information taking form.
And how did it relate to me?

I left this meeting thrilled. I suddenly had a seal of approval from someone whose judgment I trusted, because his reasoning and his methods could lead a person toward the path that suited him best in life. I received confirmation that I, me, myself alone, and not anyone else - not another doctor, not a psychologist, not another book, not another drug, not another treatment - would save me. Only I knew for sure the right track for me, the right path for me, only I could feel and know how to change… and, hence, I had the power to change!

What a huge insight. I was given back the power to take care of myself, retrieving the power to manage and control my life, which was, so far, flown and scattered. My life had been scattered among the diagnoses of doctors, therapists, medications, supplements, techniques, comments from friends, strangers and family near and far, of spouses, the whole world around me… everyone had the power on me but the only person I did not trust was myself. I wanted this sense of power once again for myself! There, I was just about to catch it, to get back the reins of my life and steer the carriage of my life to safety, to the right place for me, to where I wanted it, to a place of peace and quiet, great joy and optimal health.

WOOHOO! It was huge! It immediately changed the image of my life!

Thank you dear Lord!

Today I know that success is largely an act of perseverance and determination of the heart, at a place where others would have long given up.

I remember from my meetings with the psychologist that he believed change is the province of those who make a special effort to bring it on and that too few people are aware of the great contribution of change to the improvement of life and getting maximum pleasure and satisfaction, and that is why those who are not aware of that find it difficult to work to achieve it. His words from the past flashed through my mind like thousands of red lights. I remembered the words of the psychologist: that in order to succeed along the way, one has to practice the skills that he has not yet developed, over and over again. What were those skills? What should I develop? I had not the slightest idea, and therefore I didn't rest a single day; I searched my path through the dense forest to build myself a new future - more optimistic, better, truer and healthier.

Dreams Come True

Malcolm Fobs, an American publisher and businessman, said: "Who ceases to dream ceases to live!"
I, who previously had no real dreams other than the desire to be like everyone else – to feel no pain - felt that I wasn't alive and I so wanted to live!!!

I sat in front of the computer and visited websites to find information and ideas on different pastimes. I reviewed my skills, what I'm good at and what had interested me in the past, but had since faded with the flow of life's routine. I thought about the things I loved and knew how to do. From there, I started a personal process of research and testing and growing into other realms. Guided by the psychologist, my valued and important friend, I made a list of areas of my interest, past and present: accordion lessons, music, dance and painting. As a child, I played the accordion and occasionally danced to the beat of the sixties. And so I browsed the internet for hours, and I remembered the days when I'd attended a meditation course, which had also included painting. I couldn't draw, I'd never painted, but the painting bug had already infected me. I felt a little joy when I touched the colors. Indeed, for that class we would bring along colors, fabrics, paint brushes, cut up newspapers, and we also meditated. I loved touching the colors and creating shapes. I had done some embroidery, sewing, knitting and created art with various materials. Painting had pulled me into its lap, but I was not able to develop it because I'd always wavered between reading (dozens of books lay on the shelves in my house) and painting. Reading had always been easier. To draw, I had to set up my easel in the middle of the living room, where the space would get messy, and then have to clear up after, clean and store the equipment, just to realize the creative process… complicated and lengthy. Reading books was the easier choice - you sit down and read for as long as you can.

Up till now I had never had a corner of my own for painting or doing personal things. But the painting bug was calling me and I resolved to paint on a daily basis. I felt it would give me a sense of peace and serenity.

You could say that I chose to focus on the possibility that painting could be the new direction in my life, but, actually, painting chose me. I increasingly felt that I could devote a special part of each day to painting, for colors and shapes, feeling a kind of quiet. It seems that when we do something that intrigues us and enriches us, we disconnect from the constraints of day-to-day reality and devote ourselves to our love.

I decided to create a personal space at home, just for me. My children had grown and everyone had his own room with a TV and personal computer. I never had a place to occupy myself at home. I would always find solutions for everyone, and I never thought that I deserved a space of, perhaps, even just one meter by one meter, for my own personal use. I had never taken care of my own needs! It became clearer and sharper with each passing day, more and more, because the need for privacy was awakened in me; to have a place of my own, to sit, write, concentrate, paint and be with myself quietly, as was necessary in those days. I noticed that all of the family used all of the house, but retired to their rooms when they wanted to be alone with themselves with their business, but I was at their disposal at any given moment, and when I wanted some quiet moments, I had to shut myself in the bedroom. This was not what I wanted. I did not want to sit on my bed – a bed is designed for rest, or sleep, or to spend intimate time. I wanted to create, write, dream, think and paint. It struck me that in my own private house, my fortress, my safe space, I did not have a single area which was my own. This thought was clear and ran around in my head and would not leave me. I felt frustration, shame, helplessness and anger at everyone and especially at myself. How could I have let this situation continue for years?

Now I decided to make a change, put myself first and focus on my health, to do what was right for my body and soul that wouldn't harm others or come at their expense, of course. So far, my children, my ex-husband, my partner, my parents, my job - everyone - were first in the order of priority.

I began to consciously change my view of things and when I persevered in that, I noticed that things were slowly changing.

I decided to become an expert on fibromyalgia by "connecting to what is" in me and in my surrounding. I created a change that began with the will to be healthy, and became real by my actions.

First of all, I cut myself off from all the negative information which surrounds us for much of the day. I canceled my subscription to the daily newspaper, I stopped listening to the news and watching television programs and chose to focus on reading positive material and responding to its encouraging, funny and heartwarming subjects. I listened to relaxing music for many hours, meditation music, calming music that effortlessly transports the soul through refining processes. I would go to sleep with music and fall asleep while it was playing. If I woke up in the middle of the night, I'd replay the disc over and over. I surrounded myself with some kind of transparent bubble that contained only pleasant things that were good for me. I saw the world through the bubble I'd created and let in only what suited me. I did not allow anything that was not in my favor to come near.

I fixed myself a place in the house for the purpose of creativity, solitude and writing. I planned a space with plasterboard walls in part of the living room where I could place a small television, a computer and a wall to paint on. I'd paint on the floor and spread my colors and accessories around and be in nobody's way. Only I would go into this corner, and it wouldn't disturb the routines of the household. A few days later, the space was taking shape. I hung a plaque on the wall and shelves too, and created a space of privacy.

Seeing the new space forming was a defining moment, a moment of cognitive change. I faced it and smiled. I felt pleasant sensations surrounding my aching body and I realized I was at the beginning of real change.

I began to notice things that were happening to me and explored what led to what - what caused aggravation, and what was beneficial. I stayed away from people who were not supportive, whether they were my friends, family members or otherwise, doctors or therapists who provided no hope, and from all who made me feel bad. I stopped complaining, which was an internal decision between me and myself. If I had a complaint, I nipped it in the bud and solved it before I could start whining about it. I cocooned myself in a supportive, sympathetic, flattering and loving environment.

Albert Einstein, the father of the theory of relativity, said: "In difficulty lies opportunity."

I could already see it was the same for me.

From my experience and studies, I already possessed vast knowledge, and now a clear awareness had been added to it. I did things through awareness. I turned difficulties into opportunities to create something new that was yet unknown to me.

And so it was that while surfing the internet, I found a center for Intuitive Painting in Tel Aviv, and immediately called to find out about it. I had never let the grass grow under my feet. I arranged a meeting with the director of the center and arranged to meet him with enthusiasm and anticipation. The director of the project was a psychiatrist who founded the Center for Intuitive Painting from the idea of using "natural remedies" instead of chemical drugs, in other words, the use of art and creativity as a lever to recovery - in this case, painting. The idea was to draw freely whatever popped up in the imagination - painting that comes from the gut, without rules. Additional objectives are to reduce self-criticism, raise self-esteem and love yourself more. Thus, bit by bit, a harmonious and exquisite creation is born that makes a mark on the reality of our lives. The more creative we were, the more freedom, intense love, inner peace and self-understanding we would feel - which is what I was looking for. Noise and distraction that had intruded upon my life more in recent years were becoming unbearable and affecting my daily routine as well as my my body and soul.

And so, once a week, I would go to the center and join up with creative people and receive tuition from the instructor, paint intuitively and then spend a few minutes writing intuitively, generating an enormous release of creative energy. At no point did we learn to draw. This was actually a powerful healing process without words and without explanation, and it suppressed obsessive thoughts. All of my pain and frustrations for many years, the sorrow and the tears, poured out of me onto the canvas.

The methodology of the center was to draw a picture, then another one on top of it until we got to nine layers of paint. Thus, layers of painting, colors upon colors, slowly became a kind of harmonious and experiential magic. Though I found it hard to give up on the first painting, the temporary one, scribble on it and create a new one, this issue was a part of the healing process, during which I learned to give up, release anger and frustration and understand it was always possible to do better, to get better results... and in order to not lose what I drew every day, and because I loved the results of my paintings and I found it hard to give up on every single painting and immediately paint over it with other colors, I documented everything and took photos - one painting after another. After nine rounds of painting, I took the end result home. I framed it and hung it in the living room. The entire process leading up to the hanging of the picture gave me a feeling of liberation and immense satisfaction.

I persevered and drew at home, too, in my new space. Every time I painted for forty-five minutes to the sound of pleasant and relaxing music, I would fly into the realms of my imagination and disengage from daily events. I learned that the power of imagination is great, and if we know how to use it, our lives will be better, happier and more relaxed.

At about the same time I joined the Center of Intuitive Painting, I was approached by ASAF, a voluntary association which promotes awareness of fibromyalgia syndrome and chronic fatigue, based on the recommendation of my Ichilov support workshop guide, to volunteer and serve as the administrative director of the association, since all of the work in the association is performed by volunteers. I felt honored that, through the support workshop, I'd reached a stage of understanding about the nature of the syndrome and its implications. I wanted to contribute my humble part to the association. Since I was free most of the time, I thought that the occupation would fill my spare time, and who knew where it would lead me?

My duties included receiving membership fees, checking registration of receipts and mailing materials and information on the syndrome. I sent out letters prior to conferences, listed new members, and updated addresses.

The association supported people with fibromyalgia syndrome, promoted its recognition and provided recommendations on professional doctors and advice on such things as Social Security. This work required punctuality, diligence and perseverance - qualities which I had, and it gave me constant and independent employment activities for a few hours each day. This was often an exhausting experience because dealing with the computer and the information lists tired me. However, I felt satisfaction just from volunteering and helping others, and it was suitable for an unemployed person like me.

Losses

Six months after I retired, the relationship between my partner and I tore apart after thirteen years together. The love we felt for each other did not survive our common hardships. I suffered from severe symptoms of the syndrome, about which we'd only recently learned. They steadily worsened due to the many huge stresses which I was under: symptoms of increasing anxiety and fear, the sudden loss of ability to work, time unexpectedly on my hands that left a large void in my daily routine and the concern for my beloved man, obscure and deteriorating condition - that suffered symptoms of his own serious illness that only grew worse day by day. We did not manage to get through these difficulties together.

In a horrible and tremendously hard decision, it was decided that we would go our separate ways. I'll never forget that terrible day, the day my world was torn apart and my beautiful and united family was broken once again. Once again, I had to upset my dear parents who had suffered so much in their lives, for my sister and I and our children were the apple of their eyes and all of their concern was only for us. Once again, I had to tell them I was alone with my adolescent children. It was unbearable. I was very afraid for them. I was uncertain how they'd react, or if they would ever understand this decision. They loved my partner. Actually, I don't think there was much that could be explained. I believe they did not truly understand what I suffered from. In their later years, it was difficult for them to be considerate and understanding. They wanted us on their terms, and we aspired to fulfill their emotional and physical needs in every sense and manner. I spoke little to them about my hardships and, of course, for a long time I'd hidden my partner's illness from them. Now that there was no way to keep covering it up, I slowly began to share. Now, how was I going to explain to them what had happened?

As much as I feared for them, I didn't really care about anyone. I was in terrible mourning for myself, for my lost relationship, for my children who again saw me cry, mostly sad and dysfunctional. My days and nights were dark and I couldn't see how I was emerging from it. I only wanted the hideous pain in my body to stop, an end to the burning in my mouth, for the burning matches inside my muscles to be put out and for the heat waves that attacked me every few minutes to stop. I was a lump of pain walking on two legs. I needed tranquilizers. On the one hand, I did not like taking them, but on the other, I was in an impossible situation without them.

This couldn't be life! It couldn't be right for anyone to suffer this way! I don't deserve this! It cannot be! My brain incessantly screamed these sentences. I was a young woman in mid-life; this couldn't be all there was! I cried and cried and cried. Every now and then I relaxed, but sobs would return and attack me. I couldn't sleep, and the days and nights seemed an eternity which would not go away. I did notice, however, that the sun rose anew every morning...

When I was at the bottom of the pit, all I saw from there seemed big, intimidating and scary. I later realized that when you rise up, you are in a good place at the top, in your dreams; all things scary and threatening look small and insignificant. But at that point, I was still brokenhearted, in the depths of my suffering.

This was an important milestone. I noticed it happen every morning all over again and I remembered what Scarlett O'Hara, from the movie (which I loved) Gone With the Wind, said at the end of the film: "Tomorrow is another day!" This sentence ran through my mind over and over again. There was a little hope inside of me while I was memorizing it for myself. When I did fall asleep, it was a troubled sleep, and the mornings were the worst. I felt bad and didn't want to get out of bed. The sharp pain in my stomach, like a black hole, would not let go. I just wanted that pain to go away, but there was no pill for an aching heart. That terrible day, my heart exploded into millions of small pieces that scattered all around and away from me, tiny, luminous and elusive. My heart was one big, bleeding, and screaming sore. There was a deep void inside me, but the sun - it rose every morning anew. It was November. A chilly winter was already showing signs of arrival. My heart, cracked and broken, was frozen, but the sun shone every morning anew. That distinction brought me to where I began to think and internalize that, just as the sun rises every morning and appears among the clouds of winter, I would shine and bloom once again. This was an important goal. With no idea how it could happen, I wanted to believe in it and had high hopes for that thought.

After the harsh breakup, my mental state deteriorated further, and within a week of the day we parted, I started to suffer from episodes of dizziness that clouded my senses. Vertigo was a phenomenon familiar to me, as it is a common symptom of the syndrome. I had suffered from it every now and then. It usually took two or three weeks until it disappeared and sometimes a specific physiotherapy treatment might shorten the period of suffering.

I was totally agitated, sweat washed my body, and at night I walked between the rooms of the house, frantic with stress. I sat myself in bed and tried to relax, but the dizziness only increased. This time I was on my own and my four children were sleeping in their beds calmly and quietly, not knowing what it was all about. They themselves might have still felt unsettled by the unexpected farewell of a loved one who, for many years, had been a member of the family. How could they even begin to understand what was happening to their mother? And I just wanted to be healthy and return to normal and be the best mother in the world to them! And right now, I couldn't even think of my loved ones whom I cherished above all.

On that sleep-troubled night, I hardly slept a wink. There followed a week during which I continued to suffer with dizziness, and hoped that the spells would disappear as quickly as they had appeared. I realized that this time something different was happening and turned urgently toward physiotherapy. I had to go to the therapist in Tel Aviv who had treated me in the past. It was intolerable and inhumane because I was alone and I had no one to ask for help. I thought I could handle it by myself, since I was used to it. Two days after the treatment I had a feeling that the vertigo had eased a little, but no, it hadn't, not really. Again and again I spoke with the physiotherapist, and she suggested that I come in for another treatment. The road to Tel Aviv was a nightmare for me; tears filled my eyes as I left the apartment, and so on in the car and en route to her clinic. She was pleasant and cordial to me and comforted me with soothing words, and I felt better for the moment.

At those moments I needed support from a friend or a family member or a close girlfriend, but I did not want to bother anyone. I felt like I was complaining and whining again and again, and now I wanted to get over it myself without whining to anyone. Oh, what a mistake to make. I realized it was not good to be alone, but I paid no mind to it in those difficult moments. Stupidity or ego or failed past experience made me decide I could do it alone.

The reality of life was black. The world collapsed on top of me. I felt death staring me in the eye and inviting himself in, just as had happened to my parents during the Holocaust. I suffered pain strong enough to rip my body apart, and the horrible hot flashes had turned me into wrung-out sponge. At night I would cover myself with a blanket and draw it around me or throw it off, according to my body temperature, which rose and fell like a storm at sea. The physical therapist's treatments did not help. The thoughts that raced through my mind were terrible. Who knows what I have? What's the matter with me? What illness is wracking my body? What will happen? Who will help me?

I felt I was going crazy. One morning my condition became desperately worse, following visits to a number of professional doctors to whom I was referred for testing: a family physician, who referred me to an ENT physician, who sent me to an orthopedist who sent me to a neurologist, and so on. My son took me to Meir Hospital's emergency room, where I was examined by an ENT doctor who decided to perform extensive testing, including an MRI. That was the end of the world for me! I have always suffered from claustrophobia, so it was hard for me to face the test. The appointment was not for another two months, during which time I just existed. Fear of the examination paralyzed me. I could not get to the Center to paint due to the dizziness, and stopped leaving the house. I could barely stumble from one room to another. I stopped cooking and I found myself just lying for most of the day, unable to do anything. I could not visit my elderly parents, whose strength was spent. I could do nothing for them. This was terrible for me, and I certainly could not go and see them and to hear stories of the Holocaust and the Nazis and about the underground shelters, the murders and escapes. I'd explained to them about my anxieties and my emotional state, but they couldn't grasp it. "I can't get into the car and drive," I said, and I heard my mother weeping. It hurt me; it hurt her; it hurt us all.

My anxiety symptoms kept getting worse. From time to time, I swallowed pills recommended by the doctors, but my situation became worse. I felt like I was in a prison, behind bars, isolated from the world. Many times I felt I'd lost control, and anxiety increased my heart rate. I felt like my body was paralyzed, and was often rushed to the hospital by one of my children. The diagnosis was always the same: anxiety attack. Psychiatrists and doctors and therapists... their pills only worsened my situation. Moreover, for a long time I'd been taking a pill to lower my cholesterol and later discovered that it had side effects. A homeopath I knew explained to me that this pill could cause tremendous damage to the body and I must stop taking it immediately. He recommended that I take an alternative supplement in order to reduce my cholesterol and also advised me to change my diet. I intuitively decided to stop taking the statins. It was a decision that, later, would turn out to be correct for me.

I lay in the living room, staring, praying for help and salvation. I could not get up or move, my body was paralyzed, and the kids lived their lives around me, not realizing what exactly was going on with me.

At this point I let myself cry as much as I wanted to. I didn't care what they thought, and I didn't want to hide the grief that gripped me, or the fear of what was happening to me while suffering from the dizziness.

Thoughts in my head went back and forth – I had a relationship, I'd loved my job, I'd raised my children with dignity, I'd had a good life and was a good person. How could I suddenly be left without a job, without a partner, but with pain, sorrow and tears, unable to see myself and my future?

I remembered from the many books I read, books that brought me strength countless times, the words of Abraham Maslow, a social psychologist: "In order to change, a person has to change his awareness of himself." This information slowly permeated my brain until it became an established fact.

While waiting for the MRI test which would seal my fate, I had time to be by myself - just me and my harsh thoughts, sitting alone and thinking about the course of my life. I understood very well that things don't just happen, but I still failed to understand why my list of sufferings was so long, because I regularly suffered from some new affliction, and although I went to many doctors and psychologists following the recommendations of acquaintances and friends, there was no improvement in my condition. I had seen dozens of therapists and therapeutic counselors who used different techniques, such as homeopathy, Chinese medicine, alternative medicine, and more. I tried dietary changes and all kinds of dieting methods according to Ayurveda, Sara Hamo, by blood type and more. I refrained from eating chocolate and fatty cheeses and I didn't drink Coke or coffee. Some eased my condition, some didn't affect it at all. I also tried supplements and received recommendations for different kind of sports. I was treated in the Grinberg method for five years, and had a lot of massages. In truth, I was addicted to them as they were soothing and pleasant, taking me out of my daily routine. I tried acupuncture, but it was torture. The application of the needles, which I shouldn't have felt, was very painful for me. I was also sensitive to light, heat, moisture, cold, odors and noise, and right now my body also prickled all over. I'd tried the Alexander Technique and the Feldenkrais method, but they only helped me in the short term. The pains came back big time.

For years, especially after giving birth, I'd taken part in various classes such as exercise, yoga and aerobics, but had not persisted with them. My body collapsed, and my motivation to continue was low. I was always suffering, and I could not persevere. Walking was a torture for me, my legs hurt, and I could not stand for more than a minute. Going up or down the stairs was difficult.

From the age of twelve I had suffered from severe menstrual pains, as well as from premenstrual syndrome. Every now and again I had mouth ulcers and troublesome sores, and my mouth would feel all fired up and burned. My lips chapped so I couldn't put on lipstick, and I had allergies that prevented me wearing eye makeup. Sunlight had always hurt my eyes. I wore a hat and covered my eyes with dark sunglasses, and before I went out, I'd rub my body with sunscreen. In winter time I suffered from the cold. My fingertips, feet, hands and nose, which turned red, were always cold. Wind bothered me and burned my skin and ears. In enclosed spaces I suffered from the heat and cold alternately, requiring that I take off or put on a sweater as needed, and constantly change the temperature of the air conditioner. At the office where I'd worked, a fan blew toward me and as far as I was concerned, winter lasted until midsummer; while everyone else was wearing shorts, I was still in long sleeves.

On top of that, I couldn't stand fluorescent lights, and so where I worked, a table lamp was provided to neutralize the fluorescent light. I also refrained from entering supermarkets and various locations lit by fluorescent lights, and was unable to open drinking bottles and cans, or lift heavy packages without suffering pains in my neck and shoulders.

My pain threshold was very low. Every touch or random bump into a piece of furniture would leave a bruise at the point of impact. In between all of this, I suffered years of ringing sounds and echoes in my ears. There were times when I suffered from dizziness, but I'd learned to deal with them. The list goes on: allergies to tropical fruit, intolerance of the smell of citrus and flowers, as well as nausea near pine and eucalyptus trees and their kind. Twenty years ago, lesions started growing in my nose and every year and a half I had them removed by a Mohs procedure. In 2007, I had a big excision with an ear-nose skin graft. My mental condition was grave and I required medication for several months. I had to drink prune juice or eat bran to regulate my bowel movements, but, frankly, that did not always help.

In addition, I sometimes suffered from heart palpitations. Up to the age of thirty-five, I would use the elevator freely to get to the higher floors, but suddenly started to get anxiety attacks. Then there was the time when I sat in a cinema and waves of sweat poured over my body, and I needed a fan. Thus, I became breathless for no reason and suffered from anxiety.

Yes, I even found it hard to tear a piece of paper in half, or use scissors. My fingers become stiff and any action that involved a small amount of effort was hard for me. For years, I'd been incapable of ironing or folding clothes, and had a maid to come in to do this.

When I was diagnosed as having fibromyalgia syndrome, I received, on the doctor's recommendation, a voucher for treatments in a heated pool at Lowenstein Center. I would pack a bag with clothes, start up my car and drive to the parking lot. From there I would walk on foot to the clinic carrying a heavy bag, then change clothes and put on a bathing suit, perform the water exercises, hoping that they'd relieve the situation, dress again and go home. However, I would get home more tired than ever, so it didn't really help. On the contrary, the effort was enormous and the benefits were negligible. The pains in my body would not let me rest. For a while, my right knee hurt and I was like a disabled person, with only one useful leg. I could barely walk. I had X-rays, I went to physical therapy, and I was examined by orthopedists. I got a shot of cortisone, but nothing improved my condition. I limped for months, but carried on until eventually the pain stopped.

I thought about all these things in sequence and my soul grew even darker. What was going on here? What was happening to me, and why? What was I not seeing? What was it that I didn't understand? There was nothing I hadn't yet tried, yet nothing really helped. I lay on the living room couch with severe dizziness, dysfunctional, my heart broken, lonely, facing the white ceiling in a silent house. What now?

I want to live! I want to be healthy! I want to be happy! I have children! I have parents, I have a family, and I'm young.... I want to live!
One thought after another - but how? How to get up and go on?

Faith

"Coincidence is God's way of remaining anonymous."
Albert Einstein

On the counter in the living room was a pile of CDs. I remembered one of them, given to me two years previously by a girl I knew in the army, a religious girl I'd bumped into after not seeing her for thirty-five years. The CD was called The Heart of Things. Two years, and I'd never had time to listen to it, but I hadn't thrown it away like other unnecessary items at home.

I suddenly remembered that CD. Why now? I searched for it frantically. I looked at the cover: The Heart of Things: the big secret of the little details, disc no. 82 from the teachings of Rebbe Nachman of Brasslav, and below appeared the sentence: I am looking for myself, then below, in smaller print: for the complete healing of body and soul.

My hands were shaking as I put it in the player, and I listened to it over and over again. The CD was a lecture on stopping - stopping and looking... pausing to listen to the sounds of life... pausing and listening to the universe around you, stopping the mad daily dash and just watching and seeing. It actually was the situation that had been forced on me. I lay on the couch, my eyes fixed on the white ceiling. Someone from above had stopped the endless stream of tireless work in my life. This CD had waited for me for over two years so that I'd get it at the exact moment I needed it. Is that not observation from above? Was someone listening to me? Someone had heard my cry!

It seems that when darkness is great, you can somehow see the starlight, and I saw, I saw it indeed!

A stream of big, hot tears started to trickle down my cheeks. I let them flow like a waterfall, my heart weak and my body shuddering. I wasn't functioning. Suddenly I didn't mind at all. I lay on the sofa and looked up at the ceiling. These were pure moments of great insight descended on me from above, directed to me alone, for my ears alone, for my torn heart. Since that day I did not answer the phone for almost two months. I refused to see anyone. I turned my friends away; only my children saw me, and my sister came in to visit me. I did not go to see my parents, nor did I speak with them twice a day on the phone as usual. My sister would tell them a little about me and thus relieved me of my duties to communicate.

I sentenced myself to complete uncertainty by choice - to accept this situation and love it - a task which was totally illogical for someone like me, a sworn perfectionist, someone who must have control over everything. Usually I am observant on both the big and small things; everything must be neat and clean, beautiful and well maintained, right on, the sooner the better. I have a high level of self-discipline and self-criticism and I am hard on myself regarding getting results.

How, all of a sudden, would I give up on knowing? On clearly knowing? On any partial knowledge? Something? A lead? What was going to happen to me? Yes, I agreed to be in a state of uncertainty for as long as it took, no matter how long. I remembered the phrase, a time for everything. Apparently, it was my time, now, to lie helplessly and let time do its thing. Time goes by either way, and at that time I'd keep quiet, lie down and stare at the ceiling, as I was doing right now. This is the situation, Accept it, I said to myself, inside. Suddenly, I was not really alone. It was me and myself. I talked to myself... Quiet now! You prayed for this tranquility, you wanted it - you got it! So be quiet, enjoy the peace and that's it - just quiet. Later, we'll worry about later....

I knew that the way I went clearly allowed only one path to walk on - inside myself! I had tried other ways but found no solution in them.

I knew that I needed to deal with the syndrome and find a way to end the ills from which I suffered. I was stricken with vertigo, suffered from dizziness, my body was weak and there was not a drop of energy left in me. My heart was broken and crushed. A deep chasm opened up before me and I did not know which path to walk and where to. What would become of me and how would I rehabilitate myself and march on towards a normal life?

Inside me, along with the fragments of despair, was a streak of light - a thin strip entirely woven in my body. The strip of faith, I called it. I was always an optimistic girl. I knew there must be good in every situation, so I mustn't lose hope; there was always something more to do that hadn't yet been done. Such was I: a fighter, against all odds. Perhaps I was like my father, who never gave up even at the most difficult times, and was creative and resourceful and acted in every way to save himself and others to survive the Holocaust. Perhaps.

Yes, I was weak in mind; yes, I was weak in body. Many times I broke down, felt scared and anxious, but inside me there was the same strip of faith, standing firm.

I want to live... It was a thin and quiet whisper in my ear, inside my heart, a determined and constant whisper. I want to live, I can do it, I can do more and I want more. I won't give up. But, how?

I dug through my mind, and at times left the 'how' and I just existed. I allowed myself to hurt, to feel miserable, and be really sick, suffering, hurting and dysfunctional. I cared for nothing. I was here in the room and the whole world was running without me, and that was fine. I lost control, I gave up on it. I simply was. And that was it.

I had to go from what I knew so far into that which was unknown and hidden from my eyes. Only then, I knew, could I learn something about what was happening to me.

Does choosing faith, optimism and life against all odds, when it seemed that I had no choice because fate would choose for me, get me anywhere? I later found we have the ability to choose and make the state of victimhood an experience with a mission and purpose and knowing that we can act. I accepted the fact that there is probably more than one correct truth and, at that moment, I did not know what it was. In different conditions, we need different and contradictory images of reality. They might all be true, and therefore complement each other.

At first there was nothing I could do. In order to gain insight on what I needed to do and how, I had to choose quiet, seclusion, disappearance, silence and immobility. I sentenced myself to consciously avoid conversations that emptied me of energy and weakened my will to go on my way. And so it was that I finally gave in. I gave up, and raised a white flag.

Among the CDs of soothing music that I listened to in those difficult days, I found another important CD: Undo negative thinking. I listened to that CD over and over again… listened and internalized, and when negative thoughts came, I replaced them with others, even though I did not have a solid basis for this. I decided to scrap the thought and choose something positive. Later, it turned out to be a great technique.

I also remembered the words of one of my important mentors, who explained in one of our meetings that our minds tend to sometimes bully the natural, quiet and balanced state of man, and thus lead to a situation of isolation, emotional suppression, stress and lack of inner peace. That calmed me down a bit, because these things that sank deep into my brain in those meetings began to float in my mind that was troubled, confused and full of thoughts running inside me.

I hunted for the notes I'd written at the time on the course, to refresh my memory on the Scripture. These helped me to understand my situation.

Indeed, when a person reaches the abyss, he has the opportunity to look up and from such a low place he can either wilt, if he chooses to do nothing, or to grow and flourish.

"Do not trust your mind," said the Buddha, and his message was about awakening and liberation, once and for all, from the power struggles between our head and emotions. Don't allow control to the head, nor to emotion. Neither of them should lead. There is another character in the head, "the real self" and it is the host of the head and feeling. It is the landlord.

The inner voice can change, become much more positive and sometimes even grow silent. It's possible to change the internal atmosphere and, through the right practice, introduce tenderness and compassion in place of internal tension and struggle between the head and the emotion inside of us.

These were words I could identify with because they suited the inner desire that was in me. However, I still did not know how to get to this long awaited status. It sounded wonderful. It is possible to awaken the landlord so that he'd take responsibility - it said so in my notes - so that he would lead and go forward. This is the essence of the spiritual path in Buddhism. I liked the words at those moments. I already wanted to be in this place, to be the one leading my life, to navigate between the emotion and the mind changing and becoming compassionate and soft with myself - to resolve the internal struggle that raged within me. I realized it wouldn't happen in a heartbeat. I realized that I needed to be patient and that patience was going to be the keyword for me at the present moment and in the days ahead - to be patient with myself and with what was happening to me in the process. This insight greatly helped me to emerge from the black depths in which I was immersed.

With this patience, I felt inside me some kind of small faith that everything was in my favor and that something positive must come from the situation I was in. It seemed that faith is a drug known to achieve victory where despair is celebrating.

One day when I was sitting in the living room as usual, watching the green tree outside the window and the sun peeping into the house, I started flicking through the TV channels. I didn't have the patience to watch TV and basically nothing interested me. I wanted to keep my own silence, so I zapped through the channels rapidly. Suddenly I stopped on a channel called Karma, broadcasting various awareness programs. I had not seen it before, but now I glimpsed an image of an affable man with a white beard and a soft voice, and I realized I was watching a lecture by Rabbi Michael Laitman who headed a group at Bnei Baruch and was the head of the community for learning and spreading of Kabbalah method In The Shadow of the Ladder. I was surprised that I was getting this channel because I did not order it and hadn't paid for it. That didn't bother me - I was attentive to what I heard. The words were directed at me - every word of the Rabbi was directed to me. How does he know who I am? What was I missing? And how much I suffer? I was hypnotized. I eagerly heard every word he said and it felt like cool water given to a thirsty man in the desert. Every sentence he said touched me. Every word he said was directed at my situation, and each answer given was directed towards the questions that raced through my mind. I felt this channel was created just for me. It's a gift! I recognized it was a gift and I was very glad of it.

I felt reconnected to the stream of life once again. If at first I was unplugged then suddenly I had been plugged in again and the strip of light inside my body gained momentum and strength and stood a little taller. Suddenly I got answers to questions that bore into my mind and I knew what to do. I knew how I was going to recover. There was an insight here that brought a clear knowledge and an empowerment of inner strength. From there, it was a short path to action. Every day, from now on, I would make sure to sit for hours in front of the television with a bowl of fresh fruit and vegetables in front of me, gulping down the rabbi's words.

A week later, the channel suddenly disappeared from the screen. An invisible hand had sent me the channel, so that the rabbi's insights would reach me and allow me to recover. Not coincidence, but a guiding hand. I rushed to call the cable company to subscribe to the channel and went back to watch the rabbi, whose words acted as a cure for the wounds of the heart. I don't remember his exact words, but from the first moment that I understood what he was saying, I got answers to all sorts of questions running around in my head and everything started falling into place. What was the reason for these occurrences in my life and why did they happen to me, of all people? It was obvious that I was doing something wrong in my life and so I listened over and over to the rabbi's words, without interruption, totally focused on his words, feeling optimistic about my life from now on, realizing that anything in life can change, if we just want and believe.

I'm not staying where the pain is, because I am worthy and I can come out of this situation, I thought to myself, and cheered up a little.

In addition to the programs on Kabbalah, other programs dealt with awareness, Buddhism and people who made impressive achievements in life. Every morning, I would wake up and go to the kitchen, cutting some fresh vegetables, dabbing them with olive oil and adding two slices of whole wheat bread. I ate with pleasure. I knew that in a few minutes I'd be watching the rabbi's lectures and sink into a completely different reality of life, one uniquely experiential and unusual.

One day I threw open the window and shutters of the living room, which I had not opened for about ten years, and the sun's rays came in, warmed the house and my body, and I was holding a glass of water in my hand. I grabbed the remote and flicked to the relevant channel just in time to see Rabbi Laitman announcing that very soon a large conference would take place in Tel-Aviv, to run for three days. I immediately decided to sign up for the conference because

I was looking for other interests besides drawing. In the meantime, I'd also meet people, talk with them, I'd get to know them and maybe make some new friends. I decided that by the time of the conference I would be completely healthy, so pre-registered for the three days and I looked forward to it eagerly. But a few days before the deadline, I was still feeling sick. My mood was low and my body was hurting. I felt dizzy and constantly thought I was about to fall. I knew that I could not attend the conference as I wanted to. I contacted the conference organizers and asked if I could come for only one day, and they agreed. I informed them that I'd try to make the first day, at least. I felt like the things that were going to be heard there were important to me and may bring about a turning point in my life. I had to store more mental strength. I felt I was already in the process of change burning inside me to advance forward.

On the morning of the conference, I could hardly dress myself and literally crawled towards the car. Every movement was hard for me. The dizziness was not over yet. I felt suffocated, sweat washed my body, and my pallor was evident in the rearview mirror. I washed my face, said goodbye to my youngest son and barely managed the stairs. Luckily, I lived on the first floor and made it to the car, started the engine and began to drive. . It took enormous effort and I felt the pace of my heartbeat increasing. I wanted to give up on the conference, but I tried to think positive and told myself that the feeling would pass and when I got to the conference I'd surely feel better. I fought against my body. I fought for my life. I could not afford to give up. I drove slowly and carefully, reached the parking lot and went into the auditorium. I looked for a place to sit. The tables were labeled with names of cities in Israel, so I sat next to a woman about my age who was also from Herzliya, and we exchanged a few words. In between, I talked with other people sitting around the table and felt how pleasant it was to be around them. Moments later, the rabbi came on stage and I was excited! The morning's issues behind me for a while, and we were all thirsty to hear him.

Half a day passed and it was already noon. Lunch break was announced, but I felt I could stay no longer. I was weak and dizzy, the lights hurt my eyes and the sound of thousands of people singing, dancing and cheering was impossible for me to bear. I told the woman that I'd just met that I was going home because I suffer from vertigo and suddenly I saw a spark in her eyes. She said to me, "I work for a doctor who specializes in dizziness. Would you like to come to his clinic?" I smiled to myself and wondered about this next coincidence. A coincidence? I pulled a notepad from my bag and wrote down the phone number. I got home weak but satisfied, wiping away my streaming tears. I was thrilled by my experience and there was a new excitement in me, a budding hope, fragile and soft, along with a sense of calm and relaxation.

I followed the remaining days of the conference online. I could not leave the house. I was exhausted and weak, yet what was said at the conference strengthened my spirit. I started feeling better. I received answers to the questions that plagued my life. I decided that I must keep in touch with people I met at the conference who showered me with warmth and love. This was a group of friends worth sticking to. For years I'd taken part in group meetings on guided imagery and meditation, but here I felt new flows and new insights that gave me strength and increasing faith and a strong desire to continue to overcome my illness, my fears and my frustrations. I realized there was a connection between all the events and experiences and symptoms and feelings that had happened in my life. I realized I'd lived without awareness of what was happening around me. One thing led to another. I always responded to all kinds of stimuli - my mind was stormy and agitated and restless, and found no rest or peace. I would try to escape the suffering, but I was wasting away. I stumbled over daily tasks, almost becoming powerless. I began to realize that I could control the reality of my life, decide consciously to take responsibility for my decisions. The conference provided me with strength and leverage and a refuge from where I was at. I knew it was all up to me and my willpower. I felt my rehabilitation process had already started and it was just a matter of time until I would be completely healthy.

Disillusionment

Of course, there was no possibility of any action befor I began to realize that something needed to be done.

But from that moment of recognition, dozens of paths and courses of action opened up before me.

A deep insight got into my new way of thinking, into the deep tunnels of my subconscious: every desire has the right to come true, because if I could not achieve it, I would not want it in the first place! And although I experienced serious and unpleasant health issues with strange and restrictive physical feelings, I deserved - and could achieve - good health, healthy physical sensations and a happy body. This was my decision: that what I wanted was my dream!

I wanted to bring live energy to my body that would cancel the statistics and ignore the intellect and the circumstances and what everyone around me was saying. I wanted to believe it was possible for me to create a different life.

I decided that I wanted to be healthy. I remembered reading in a book by Napoleon Hill that those who succeeded in life started on the left foot (i.e. badly) and underwent many heartbreaking struggles before reaching their target and that no one is ready for something unless he believes he can get it, and that there must be faith, not only desire and hope. I already had hope, desire, faith and a strong will to be healthy and therefore I made an appointment with the homeopath recommended by my new friend from the conference. Following an extensive examination, he wrote down a long list of supplements I should take. He claimed that my body needed them because it was empty of vitamins and minerals. All the resentments, frustrations and disappointments had hit me badly and emptied my body's vital reservoirs, so it needed the supplements in order to recover and return to normal.

When I got home, I was hit by a strong anxiety attack, felt dizzy and wanted to vomit my very soul. The dietary supplements in my bag frightened me. I couldn't predict their effect and had to face the fact that they might worsen my condition, as had often happened in the past. I had always taken pills of one sort or another and they had not always been kind to me. I rang my sister to share my conflict. I was in a state of terrible anxiety. My sister hurried round and immediately contacted the homeopath who simply told her that I needed to take the dietary supplements if I wanted to get better.

A few minutes later my sister came back to me and insisted I take the pills. "You have no choice. If you want to get better, you have to take the supplements like the doctor said. You have to trust someone and if you had enough trust to consult him, then stick with the treatment. What's the worst that could happen? These are natural supplements. Believe you'll get better!" My sister tried to dissolve my anxiety and promised she'd stay with me. Suddenly I remembered my decision to trust in my recovery and remembered that I had to dispel my old fears and have faith that it was possible for me to be healthy. I started taking low doses of supplements so that my body would get used to them: vitamins D, B, magnesium, seaweed and more.

Slowly, my dietary habits changed. Every morning I would chop fresh vegetables, slice whole wheat bread, take the food supplements and drink a lot of water. I stopped using my usual products and started consuming wheat flour, brown rice and brown sugar. I cut down on sweets and tried to think positively. I recognized obsessions and immediately replaced those thoughts with other, better ones, like those I read in my books. I put empowering faith into my inner speech: It is possible for me to live in optimal health!

I realized that there was no limit to what I could be, do, or achieve, except the boundaries that I set for myself and those I could expand. That's where I was headed.

The food supplements I got from the homeopath started to make a positive impact. I decided to take another step towards my recovery - bodily movement. Every day I made sure to get out and walk moderately. On the first day I walked 100 yards and got home feeling weak. On the second day I walked for 200 yards and then 300. My legs were heavy, my body swayed and moved with discomfort. The dizziness still hadn't let go of my head, but I did not give up. My lungs were filled with fresh air and I forced myself into one directional thinking: while walking moderately, I repeated out loud to myself: This action promotes my health... All that I do is for my personal gain... I'm growing stronger by the minute... Every cell of my body is vital, healthy and full of joy... and so I slowly felt better. Every day I increased my modest route and went home to watch the wonderful lectures on TV. Besides the rabbi's lectures on Kabbalah and the Zohar, which were fascinating, there were also programs on awareness, healthy diet, changing lifestyle habits, exercises in Chi Kong and Tai Chi, and interviews with people who had been laid so low that their lives had collapsed but had recovered. I sat and told myself: If they can do it, so can I! I drew inspiration and strength from them, while I kept reading my awareness books and grew stronger by the day.

It was clear to me that the world is what I think of it. It was clear to me that I see the world through my eyes and with my own interpretation, but the most important virtue is the ability to learn both from my personal experience and from the experience of others, insights I got on the way to healing.

Over time I walked longer distances. It was bliss to walk in the park and look around me with alertness, giving thanks for creation. I walked and carefully examined my surroundings. I talked to myself and said out loud, "Here is a tree," and, "There's a bird flying," "Here's some green grass," and, "There's a bright blue sky." That was a technique I used to make myself stay in the moment, without escaping to my usual thoughts. With every moment, I thanked the Lord for putting me back on my feet and letting me enjoy this beauty around me. The days when I lay helpless, dizzy and in pain were still fresh in my mind so I thanked the good Lord for giving me strength not to give up and for getting me out of the darkness into a place of light and beauty. I got back to drawing a little after a long break due to my physical weakness and I also met with the psychiatrist and the director of the Center for Intuitive Painting. There had been an improvement in my condition after the Kabbalah conference and taking up painting again, but I was still not feeling completely well. The psychiatrist gave me some cognitive exercises to practice at home. I bought a book he wrote on the subject, "A Moment Before the Psychiatrist" and again I thought about how I was not going to give up and how I wanted to continue fighting for a better quality of life. And so, every day, I would shut myself in my new tiny room, close the door and write notes in the book and practice according to the guidelines. This book was intended to help those who want to come out of depressive illness and to make a difference in their lives, and to provide an opportunity for self-healing instead of going to a psychiatrist. It helped to convert the need to take pills into actions more natural to the body, into creativity and positive thinking, allowing them to cope with the difficulties of reality by himself. And so I would regularly write in the book, trying to meet my task and decision to live without visiting doctors and without the need for expensive treatments.

The book occupied me for a few months and so I contacted my intuition, connected with myself, controlled my mind and felt new blood flowing in my veins. I realized that I was on the right path and on my way to a happier life, more joyous, and of better quality. All along, I continued to watch the Kabbalah programs on television and draw additional strength. I also signed up for a virtual forum with delegates of the conference, from whom I received reinforcement, support and endless encouragement.

He who learns must suffer. And even in his sleep, pain that cannot forget falls, drop by drop, upon the heart, and in our own despair, against our will, comes wisdom to us by the awful grace of God.
Aeschylus

At this point my body started growing stronger and I knew in my mind that I had to capitalize on the healing already achieved. I wanted to feel an internal rejuvenation of my abilities in order to create things with a lot of enthusiasm and vitality. I still did not feel it, but I felt that it should happen.

All along, I persevered with drawing for at least an hour a day, and I read dozens of important books which gave me hope and strengthened my belief in my abilities and my strength. I read about people who'd had bad experiences, who with the force of one decision, determination and perseverance, were able to change their lives, reverse the processes that led them downhill and ride their success as they had dreamed, planned, deserved, and were able.

I, too, made such a decision. If there were people who succeed, I could too. I also wanted to succeed and I'd do whatever it took to make that happen. If imagination was their most powerful weapon and every day they imagined that they were in a different reality, a successful, optimistic and hopeful one, and did activities that promoted them towards their target - so could I. If there were people who could succeed and do it to the best of their abilities, so could I. I wanted to succeed, too! These thoughts raced through my mind. It became increasingly clear to me that there was a price to pay and that I was ready and willing to pay it in order to succeed. I'd do whatever it took, whether it was to sit at home and read books, highlighting the important things in the Scriptures and memorizing them, or diligently performing them. If I could not complete all of my tasks in a day, I'd do better the next. I wouldn't give up until I got the result I wanted. This was my decision. Firm and stable, stronger than me, the decision to be healthy flowed through my body and blood and circled my head over and over again. I knew inside my mind that much of my future was already inside me, but I also knew that I did not know how to achieve it. I had to continue to ask questions and seek new avenues for learning and development. I gave myself up to something unknown.

In order to achieve my goal, I bought a large notebook and sat down to write in it as recommended by the author Julia Cameron in her works "The way of the Artist" and "Riding the Dragon" and according to the "way of the the Artist" workshop I experienced two years before. I intuitively wrote whatever came to my mind. Each day, I diligently wrote the sentence: What is my dream?

I did not know how to answer myself, except that I wanted to be healthy. I wrote about my desire to get well, to stop whining and complaining. I wanted to be strong, healthy and happy – yes, to be happy seemed like a worthy cause. Healthy and happy. But how to do it? What did it mean? The needs of my mind versus my body's ability presented a huge gap to bridge.

I continued to write according to the recommendations in the book. I made a list of all the good things in my life and suddenly I realized that there were so many of them. I started to write on paper all that I had in my life: four good kids, a house and a car, parents still living and always with me - and at my age that was a privilege - supporting me, even if they didn't understand me. They provided me with confidence. I had my extended family, warm and loving, even if they, too, didn't understand me... It was okay, I suddenly realized I did not have to be understood. It was more important that I understand myself. Who am I? What do I have? How much I respect myself with what I had? I'd had a wonderful job that would pour a good pension into my bank account for life. I'd had two spouses who loved me for many years, even though the relationships didn't survive. We remained in good relationship till this day.I had friends who were good in heart and soul, even though they didn't understand what I was suffering of. I painted and loved it. I had a psychologist, an excellent friend. I'd had an amazing and supportive mentor for years, and in my path I encountered wonderful, spiritual teachers and all of them taught me a lot. I had great books to help me… and so on. I listed all the good things in my life, noting that until now I'd taken these things for granted, paying no attention to how, why and what things were happening.

I was already acquainted with the world of the Kabbalah by chance and when I started to write things down on paper they suddenly became tangible and numerous. I had a great faith that developed, as the days passed, into an insight from which came enormous gratitude, from the bottom of my heart toward the sky, toward the universe, toward the Creator, toward the wonderful nature around me, toward the same higher power whose existence I suddenly felt while noticing the laws of nature that whispered in my ear all along. I remembered that in my hardest and most terrible days, not too long ago, when I was in great distress, the sun showed her face to me every morning, warming my heart and giving me hope. I remembered that the harsh winter I'd come through with dizziness and cold in my heart had turned into a blossoming spring and that summer was upon us... I observed the natural laws at work, so precise, and I asked myself: What does it all say to me? And is it really so? Is it possible that I'm outside of this circle? Can I - should I - get back into it? And how do I do that? And what is this "fibromyalgia" that has plagued me throughout my life with varying levels of severity, according to what is happening around me? The answers were not long pouring out of me and went straight onto the paper.

To all the things I wrote, I added a deep gratitude for all that I had and all that surrounded me. And from there the road towards prayer - and requests from our maker, from the infinite intelligence I recognized, from a divine force that I believed existed - was a short one. I prayed for help, for guidance and advice on my new path. Of course I did not settle for prayer alone because I had realized something H U G E!

And what was this something? The same insight that changed the course of my life which was already accelerating toward change?

I realized that if I was ill and in need of treatment, no treatment in the world would ever succeed if I profited from this disease. If I profited, I would continue to be sick. The question was - what profit did I get from fibromyalgia? How did it serve me? What protection did it provide me with? And why? These questions led to many answers.

The truth is that only when I accepted myself as I am, only then could I change, only then could I bring about a change, an internal change, in my being.

This was not evasion, or indulgence, or whining. The suffering was real. The stresses and strains that I lived with were enormous. The effort I expended was unreasonable. The desire to overcome them was immense. My sensitivity guided my life, but the denial was irrational. I suddenly knew that everything I'd felt throughout the years was true and that I was born with a certain identity and must learn to accept it and not fight it. There was certainly no need to prove to others that I was the best. I simply accepted myself and made peace in my heart. It would take a long time to overcome years of ongoing frustration and denial, but now I realized that I must acknowledge that fibromyalgia was a part of me. I must love it, pay attention to it, and accept it as it was. The question was - why did fibromyalgia come to me? Why did I choose fibromyalgia?

I understood then that my fibromyalgia was meant to keep me safe, to protect me. It came for my own good all those years ago, when I could not deal with experiences and life events until I had the right tools.

I had to protect myself instead of learning and growing when the world around me flooded me. My sensitivity had made me cautious, my over awakening had caused me constant distress.

My former worldview had prevented me from discovering my full potential. My thoughts took over and came at the expense of emotional, intuitive, spiritual and healthy awareness. There was no balance between them. My intuition was blocked by beliefs I had absorbed. My fears controlled me, and stress and strain were deafening my inner voice. I could not listen to my inner voice . I could not identify the source of the problem that was hiding behind the story I told myself (you can not...you are worthless...you are not like everyone else...). So, yes, fibromyalgia had protected me, made me acknowledge my body and soul, but back then I could not see it. Now it was calling me to come back to life. Yes! Yes!

For me, Fibromyalgia meant waking up to life!

Waking Up to Life

I suddenly noticed everything around me - the leaves on the tree that stood outside my window looked greener in my eyes, the sun was more pleasant and caressing, and the sky was colored in varying shades of blue, both dark and light, and I noticed these changes. I noticed changes throughout the day. Even the seat on which I sat regularly took on an all-new meaning. I watched the endless spaces of the sky and saw the distant horizon with its strong and changing colors and I felt that I, too, had infinite spaces in me. I, too, had infinite possibilities, just like the never ending giant sea, sometimes stormy and sometime relaxed, like me, and the water still licked at the beach again and again. A small joy that pervaded me began to grow every day as a result of new insights, with new and fascinating observations, with deep silence penetrating every limb of my body. I felt like I was getting wings, like I was starting to grow and flourish. A little joy crept into my heart more and more by the day. A great curiosity made me want to know what was happening at any given moment, what I was seeing, and what it meant to me. What did it signify for me? I realized that there is meaning to life, that my existence had meaning and that I had to do something.

My rehabilitation was at full strength. I felt I was healing, that I was connecting with myself, with my inner self, which I needed and wanted to be with, none of which depended on anyone on the outside or anything material around me or external to my body. I realized what I had read so many times in the books, and I felt what I had heard from my spiritual teachers. You could call it a revelation.

It was clear to me that writing, praying and confessing were not enough. Action was necessary, but not like before. Not to be busy doing things, but being things, experiencing them, understanding them and giving them expression, creating what I know - to make my feelings and experiences into actions.

It was not too late for me to be all I wanted to be. With this feeling I continued on my way.

I went online again, looking for information about my symptoms, diseases similar to fibromyalgia, methods of healing and treatment, food, nutritional supplements, pills and their side effects, sports, music and its influence, the muscles and the way they operate, Chinese and Indian Medicine, and especially people who'd come through difficult situations. I looked for what they did, how they managed it, what strengthened them, what brought them success and I asked myself what do I need to do in order to get myself fully healed?

The MRI result was completely normal. I was very relieved. There was no evidence whatsoever of anything wrong in my head, so I concluded that the origin of the dizziness was a result of vertigo attached to my gloomy mental condition during a difficult period in my life when my body was weak and my immune system was shaky.

I went and found a renowned physical therapist who was an expert on vertigo. Within two effective treatments and after parting with a serious sum of money - but knowing that this was worth it to achieve my purpose - the dizziness passed. Of course, by that time I was regularly taking supplements given to me by the homeopath (remember how I was afraid to take them?) which strengthened my immune system. I made sure to practice the balance exercises recommended by the physical therapist, and so my balance grew stronger and I was back to my usual self.

Recovery and Fulfillment

When the dizziness stopped, I was able to connect to the Internet again. Now, much of the pain and the sadness, the loss and sickness were behind me. From all I've now done and read, I realize that I needed to get out of my comfort zone if I wanted real change. I already learned that faith, perseverance and enthusiasm support a successful change - and I longed for change.

I cannot have two identities, I thought to myself. To be suffering from a syndrome and healthy at the same time is impossible. I must ask myself what I really want. It was clear to me that action was required to attain my chosen goal, but as long as I didn't know what I really wanted, there was no chance of starting. I sat in front of my special notebook and wrote thousands of lines and from those thousands of lines, listening to music, watching the awareness channel on TV and reading books, I highlighted sentences that were important to me and I felt connected to them through that solitude that I subjected myself to. From all the insights I brought forth during that period of introspection came twelve important lines. Each named what I wanted to achieve.

This important piece of paper was something I studied several times a day and I memorized it. My mind was now flooded with ideas. I'd repressed them throughout the years just because I had no idea how to fulfill them and because of symptoms that hindered me. From the moment I wrote my important lines, which detailed clear, specific and exciting goals for me, a kind of spark was ignited in me that gave me the energy and the passion to act. I had no doubt of my ability to realize my goals. I did not know how I'd do it, but I've learned over time to ask for help and so I looked for anyone who could guide me on my way and support me. I discovered that when I ask for help or support, there's a response. Another insight - how simple it is to ask for help.

"A happy person is the one who has a dream and a goal and is willing to pay the price required to practically fulfill them."
Leon Sonos

Out of desire to promote my painting and improve my skills, I looked on the Internet for suitable options. By chance I found a site where you can upload paintings for free. I opened a page in my name and started uploading photos of my paintings. One day I was approached by an exhibition curator who offered me the opportunity to participate in a group exhibition. It sounded wonderful. Someone was interested in my work of art! I agreed, of course. I went with my family to the opening of the exhibition and I was very excited. Afterward, the desire to put on my own exhibition, just for my paintings, was born. I embarked upon this project when I was not at my best, but this new venture generated new blood in my veins. It gave me a reason to wake up in the morning and made me wake up cheerful and fresh. The activity around the exhibition, the publicity, the invitations to family and friends, hanging the works in the gallery in Jaffa - all these provided me with immense joy. The excitement was at its peak and the opening night was special and pleasing for me and my family, who could see how I was now recuperating and healing. Despite the fact that I was still sad over my broken heart of eight months earlier, I could see and understand that good things were happening to me and that I was on the right track for rehabilitation and recovery. The entire time, I made sure to keep the psychologist - my dear friend - informed. I enjoyed his support and was encouraged every time he expressed his wonder at my progress. I remembered my promise to myself to "show him" and I was proud and happy I had. This goal was a very powerful motivator for me. He could not have known how motivated I was, that time he foresaw a gloomy future for me if I will not find contentment and interest, and a means of positive self-expression.

This exhibition led to many more. I shared with the world what my hands are capable of, what I could create from my intuition, from my gut, from my pain and suffering, which had now been transformed into joy and happiness. Many who saw my paintings said that they had a healing energy. Their eyes revealed an experimental, exiting powerful world. Their warm responses brought me happiness and filled my heart with joy and thanksgiving.

If you want to see the healing process I went through with my paintings, please visit: www.talorgallery.com

"A sound mind in a sound body, is a short, but full description of a happy state in this world."
John Locke

At this point, I still suffered from a phenomenon that was tremendously troubling to me - mouth burns. For years, my palate had occasionally started to burn. No solution was found. My lips would sting and, sometimes, peel. I used creams prescribed by different doctors and took pills, but nothing helped. I was used to suffering with this and having no sense of taste. The burning pain wouldn't let go of me. I saw the best oral health doctors and they all said the same - this was another manifestation of fibromyalgia. However, my friendly homeopath recommended replacing my silver fillings with white fillings. There was a concern that these fillings were associated with mercury gas which is toxic to the body, hence the burning sensation in the mouth. This was a rather delusional theory that had its critics among the medical profession, but my despair left me with no other option but to try this too. What did I have to lose, apart from a few thousand shekels? I did it, and six months later, I'd changed almost all the fillings in my mouth. And, indeed, one day the phenomenon ceased. One step further on the way to recovery.

An article published about Dr. Ailine Aron in a newspaper brought me another step towards recovery. Dr. Aron, from the United States, had written a book called "The Highly Sensitive Person", which was yet to be translated into Hebrew. The thing that stirred my heart and turned my worldview of myself and of fibromyalgia upside down, was information about how to identify a particular feature in those of us with fibromyalgia, a feature of hypersensitivity. According to Dr. Aron, it is natural to occasionally feel that we are inundated with too much environmental stimulus, but in hypersensitive individuals it happens constantly - it's a fact of life. And if this feature stands out for us, she teaches in the book how to harness it to our advantage in everyday life. In the book she deploys her extensive experience as a researcher and as a therapist in order to help us understand ourselves and the features inherent to us, so that we may live a full and complete life.

This new insight rocked my world. This wonderful feature called hypersensitivity allowed me to intelligently consider anything with a strong intuition that I knew existed within me; a quick understanding, a reasoning and speed of response, before others had even realized what was going on, and more... Indeed, these were things I'd experienced all my life. This knowledge I now had of this wonderful feature, showed me that it's actually a gift after all, but that great sensitivity had also brought suffering when I did not realize that I was being overwhelmed with stimuli. That's why my suffering increased if I did not act properly to mitigate the rate of stimuli washing over me.

"Don't forget to love yourself."
Soren Kierkegaard

From that point on it was a short and quick road to looking at myself in a positive way, to looking at the experiences I had been through in life with a positive take for the development of higher self-esteem. I stopped pushing myself to the edge of my abilities in every perspective of my life. When the book reached the stores, I bought it at once and read it eagerly, shocked and moved by what I read. The features fitted with who I was, with the phenomena in my life. The tips and guidance in this book, brought me to a high point of view in my life. I discovered a great compassion towards myself. I discovered a great love for who I once was and for who I am today. I've forgiven myself for everything I was and for who I have become following the terrible suffering I've experienced and the different hardships that struck me occasionally in my life. I loved myself as a child, as a teenager and as an adolescent. I loved myself as a woman, as a wife and as a mother of children and loved myself for the partner I had been with my spouses. I discovered who I was then, the things I did not like about who I was, and how I'd lacked compassion for myself. Who could have felt compassion towards me back then, when I underestimated who I was and what I did despite the syndrome and the symptoms? I had not appreciated what I had. Now came a time of understanding, a time of great forgiveness, great compassion for myself, and love. It expanded from there to my environment. I forgave my partners, forgave my children who did not understand, forgave my co-workers who, for years, did not give me any credit. I forgave my former friends who'd abandoned me when I was in need, forgave my neighbors who'd bullied me sometimes, forgave everything I had not understood before. I became softer, more relaxed and appeased. I decided to put the past, along with its difficult and good experiences behind me and carry on my way.

One by one I noticed that there is no coincidence in life. There are only the things we pay attention to. When we are attentive to what's happening around us, we develop discernment.

At that time, I came across a remarkable woman, a Kabbalistic numerologist. While chatting with her, she asked if I'd ever thought about changing my name. I replied that I did not particularly like my name. I was named Tova (good in Hebrew) after my deceased paternal grandmother who perished in the Holocaust. Obviously, I was proud to be named after my grandmother, but a name is always binding, isn't it? The question, "Are you really good?" was repeated each time I introduced myself to a stranger. "Of course I'm good. I'm even very good," I would reply proudly with a smile. Yes, I later realized that I was good to everyone, except to myself. It was in my blood. I paid dearly for putting everyone before me in order of importance, while I... I considered myself last; I was at the bottom of the ladder. I realized that, too, during my recovery.

It would seem that her question about my name fell on attentive ears. A great joy awakened in me when thinking about adding to the name Tova – having a new name. I did not think twice. My intuition immediately said yes. From a list of several names she wrote down for me, the name "Talor" sprang first before my eyes and I fell in love with it immediately. (Tal = dew + OR= light, brightness).

I knew I wanted a whole new identity for myself, both in terms of the new person I'd become and in terms of the important decisions that I wanted to implement in my life at the time I first started to recover. A new name would validate my new identity. I did not drop my previous name. It had served me for many years, and I thank my parents for choosing it. Indeed, I went through all the correct procedures required to change my name, including getting the blessing of my rabbi and announcing my new name to all of my acquaintances, my family and to my dear parents. I knew that only after I informed everyone would the new name become official. My parents were very understanding. Later, I learned that my mother used my new name to tell others about me. My parents kept calling me Tova, however, and I understood their habit, after all, at their age, it was too much to demand they start calling me Talor.

Miraculously, this name brought a lot of light into my life. Everyone who heard it was very excited and it provided me with wonderful energies.

It turns out that if we devote ourselves to our vision, more and more things start to take shape and success appears from everywhere.

After my blessed recovery from the dizziness, changing my name, the renewed connection to myself, the new diet, the daily walk, taking the dietary supplements and all the other steps I took on the way to full recovery - came a desire to break the cycle of loneliness I had unwillingly sentenced upon myself. I'd shielded myself from what was going on outside for a long time. I'd abstained from friends, family and from cultural activities which I so loved in my life. Now I felt a desire to connect to this world.

One night I dressed up, put on a little makeup and went to a dance club that played music from the sixties. When I'd read about it a few days before in the newspaper, I realized immediately that I had to go there, no matter what - but would I really be brave enough to go to a club by myself? It wasn't easy at my age, after many years of being in a relationship. How would I do this? I decided to take the plunge. What's the worst that could happen? What did I have to be ashamed of?

"You must do the things you think you cannot do. "

Eleanor Roosevelt

That evening was significant in the further development of my life. Two important things happened: the minute I got on the dance floor, an ancient life force woke inside me. A massive influx of energy that had been left unfulfilled for many years burst out of me and I felt like a breeze on the dance floor! I wasn't perfectly healthy yet, but the new wind blowing through my body gave me an unfamiliar strength. I was careful not to overdo it, but I knew that my childhood dream - to dance - would be fulfilled now, and in order to dance the way I wanted to, I should find the way to full recovery.

The second thing was that I met a new friend who, in days to come, would become a soul mate. When she asked me what I did, I told her I was a painter, and that I was already retired and my main occupation today was as an artist. She immediately connected me with a well-known professional website - a networking organization for business people - and I did not understand what she was talking about, but the next day I visited it using the URL she sent me. I was very curious about everything I came across. I joined the networking group, began to attend group meetings, to meet business owners, learn how to do business, how to present myself and my occupation in sixty seconds and generally meet fascinating people in various occupations. My life was occupied and filled with interest and my time began to be filled with business meetings. Within three months I was invited to serve as chairman of a group. My organizational potential was recognized and I was offered the role, which was voluntary, but generally challenging. I hesitated because I knew I should not take on too much, but I wanted to embrace every opportunity that came my way, so I agreed to take the respected job.

That was the second time I had engaged in volunteer activities in the community. At first I'd served as administrative director of the ASAF Association, and now I was chairman of group networking meetings. During this process of getting my life back, I realized how much helping others can promote one's own health.

When you have something to give, it is worthwhile and important to do it. Giving, in itself, creates enormous satisfaction for the provider. Furthermore, there are so many benefits in the activity itself, such as getting to know people, understanding different processes and learning, day by day, about life. The very act promotes the other in at least equal measure as yourself. Therefore, for a year-and-a-half, I persevered in the fascinating role of group chairman. This occupation required interaction with people and utilized my skills. I really enjoyed the role.

Opportunities come across the person who is present, or as Jackson Brown, Jr., an American rock singer and musician, said: "Opportunities dance only with those found on the dance floor." I loved his statement. I could imagine it in my head.

In parallel with my post as group networking chairman, I continued to concentrate on painting. I participated in exhibitions and I formed a group for meditation and guided imagery at home. Meditation helped me to relax and had enabled me to fall asleep easily for many years. Poor sleep - multiple awakenings and difficulty falling asleep –had sabotaged my body many a time in the past. I was introduced to meditation as an aid in 1995. A charming mentor had worked with me for many years and now I felt I could pass this on to others. I would open the networking group meetings with several minutes of meditation. People loved coming to the group and loved to open the meeting this way. I received a lot of compliments and started to write meditations by myself throughout the year. That year I met a woman whose profession was sales and marketing and I learned from her for a while. The idea of combining meditation and fibromyalgia came to mind, and so the meditation and guided imagery CD "The Inner Peace" was born. The production process of the CD connected me with other artists. I became aware of processes that were not previously within my scope of interest. I met fascinating people and the whole process excited and moved me.

I recorded the CD in a studio with live instruments and musicians. The music was composed especially for me in a style scientifically studied by medical institutions and proven to boost healing and relaxation. I wrote the meditation and then recorded it alongside the musicians. The CD gives people in pain a personal tool to deal with various pains in the body and with impaired sleep, by themselves, naturally, without having to use any pills. It was a great success and I felt great satisfaction when its production process was completed.

Every such project in which I took part was another bright stepping stone on the road to my full recovery and rehabilitation. I felt myself getting stronger by the day and saw how creativity brought a positive energy flowing through my body and made me get up every morning feeling refreshed and full of enthusiasm for the meetings, lectures, gallery events and awareness workshops. All of these filled my day, while the evenings were often occupied dancing with my girlfriends, whose number has increased over the years. A lot of joy, vitality and great happiness in the small things embraced me. I felt how I was changing on the inside, how from a woman wracked by unexplained suffering, I had become a creative woman, expressive in every sense and manner, appreciated, loved, taking initiative and managing life according to my abilities without being ashamed.

How active am I every day? Exactly, exactly as much as I can! As much as I feel I can. No more!

I let go of the need to be like everybody else, the moment I realized how my sensitivity makes me unique and takes place in my life. Many emotional and physical phenomena disappeared from my life with no guiding treatment, I grew stronger both physically and mentally, and with each passing day I witness another breakthrough. Each time I dare a little more, and if I can't - simply let go. I no longer have the need to prove something.

I checked and asked myself: am I healthy yet? Because being healthy means living without symptoms. Don't I have any symptoms? Of course I do - all kinds, like everyone has occasionally. If so, what have I achieved? The outcome is that I have recovered.

For what is recovery? Recovery is using ability and strength to build a new life. If so, I can declare with certainty that I am healed! I am functioning at my maximum capacity with an optimistic sense of health, quality of life, happiness and contentment.

Designation

"Your duty is to find out what is the labor you must do and then surrender to it with all of your heart."
Buddha

I kept up my daily writing and introspection along with my various occupations and every now and then the question arose in me: is this my designation? Is this my dream? Is this what I want?

What is designation? I did not understand what it encompassed. What is the meaning of the word? What am I supposed to feel? The more I persisted reading the books that strengthened me, the more this word came back again and again in different variations, and one day I found the answer. This is it: it's not being a painter, it's not being a banker, and it's not studying teaching or education, nor guiding meditations. That's not it. It's something deeper, more important, something of value to humanity, to the community - to others.

Over the years, people would consult with me on different matters. More and more, people were becoming interested in why I retired from the bank. What did I do? What did I go through? And how did I recover? I realized that I was giving people answers from the bottom of my heart, answers that contained a lot of personal knowledge, life experience and wisdom gained from personal learning, from taking an interest and curiosity. All this led me, throughout all of my life, to the wonderful place where I am today. I realized that I could help people who suffer from chronic pain and sleep deficiency, as well as hypersensitive individuals with fibromyalgia syndrome and chronic fatigue. I was there. I found the way out of it. I lived through it. I beat it.

I began to appear in the media. Articles were published about the syndrome and how I wanted to help and support people, to guide and advise them from my experience of going from a state of illness to recovery. And what is recovery? The use of my abilities, skills and strength to build a good, happy and meaningful life. I was interviewed on television, by local newspapers and L'Isha magazine for women, and also on the radio program The Good Life. Now, people who sought a solution that did not involving drugs or conventional medicine started calling me - individuals looking for someone who would listen and support; someone who had been there; someone experienced who understood their language; a person who had recovered. That's me. Today, I experience great happiness and satisfaction when I help others. That's it. I found my calling. I found my designation. I started to give lectures and tell everyone willing to listen about fibromyalgia. I stayed on course in the networking site and focused on the publication of my specialty on the subject.

Fibromyalgia made me pick myself up to reach a place of spiritual and practical development and of internal and essential change.

I haven't taken any pills for years now. I make sure to take supplements and change them from time to time and I've learned to eat mostly healthy food. I changed my diet slowly. I was not extreme. Occasionally, I would read something interesting and try it to see if it suited me. I don't eat any dairy products or cheese any more, only products from goats, or sheep's milk, and I try to enrich my morning and evening meals with fruit and vegetables. Recently I came across a book about the 'green' diet and quickly implemented the recommendations. I make a green shake containing green leaves, vegetables and green fruits. This further adjustment in my diet improved my cholesterol readings. I am not extreme or strict with myself; I occasionally drink a good cup of coffee at the coffee shop, and eat chocolate or ice cream, too. The change is in the amount and in attention to what suits my body and fits the needs of my health, in being attentive and aware, not out of penance or sacrifice. I changed my eating habits and my quality of life changed with them.

Today I am a brisk and active person. I manage to do more than many others my age. Yet I know my limits well and I will not cross them. No what ifs... for example, I set several tasks for a certain day and if, ultimately, I feel that it's just too much for me, I change the order of my day or cut back on a task. I will not consume my energy. On the contrary, I listen to my body and provide it with the rest it needs. I know when to give up and how to combine dancing, walking, participating in one workshop or the other and the routine tasks of life and any other activity I set my mind to. There were times when I did not know my limitations - and I was therefore damaged physically or mentally, but now – no more!

"It is a painful thing to look at your troubles and know that you, and no other, have brought them on yourself."
Sophocles

The desire to dance continued to call me, so I took salsa lessons for a while, and then I started to learn the Argentinian tango. Tango music was often played in my parents' house. My father, who was blind in his old age, used to listen to music for hours and I would sit next to him, listening too, and change the discs for him. My love for dancing and music have now come into realization too.

"Music has a charm to soothe a savage breast, to soften rocks, or bend a knotted oak."
William Congreve

In June 2011, a year-and-a-half after accepting the role of chairman at the networking site, I closed the group and its members dispersed among other groups. I felt I should dedicate more of my time to my parents, especially my father, whose strength was waning. I wanted to be with them as much as possible as their need for my sister and me grew.

In August 2011, my father passed at the age of ninety-two. Old, tired and worn out, slowly letting go of his surroundings, he fell into the world of truth. Three months later, in November, he was joined by my dear mother who was ninety years of age. She could not and would not live without my father, whom she had known all her life.

Their death left a large and longing void in me. I was now left alone, an orphan whose mother and father who had both been strong, sturdy and supportive to me throughout my life, even though - until their very last day - they did not understand my affliction. In their own way they had lavished me with great love and paid for many of the treatments I had to go through when I was alone without a spouse and when my financial situation was dire. Still, I gratefully accepted the fact that my parents were separated from me at a time when I had got back on my feet. I thus realized that the heavens allowed me to continue my life from a place of strength. My path in life had led me to a point where I had to learn to deal with being alone, to change my way of life, to build up my spine. This change had eventually brought back my self-confidence and led me to be who I am today. Parting from parents is a part of life and isn't easy. It is sad, final and hard to grasp, but I came upon that part of my life from a conscious place, a place of acceptance and reconciliation, a place of faith, and I accepted their deaths with love and gratitude. There is no doubt that without the rehabilitation I had undergone in the previous three years, I would not have managed this bereavement the way I did.

Recovery and success: to appreciate what's good and beautiful in the world and find the good in others; be better; find a calling and stick with it knowing I eased the life of even one person.

The road was not easy, but "giving up" was not in my vocabulary. I realized that there is always room for improvement and that's what I do today. There is great satisfaction to be had in gaining abilities and being able to express them in the reality of life. There is satisfaction to be had in enjoyable and loved work, which dispels tensions. Therefore, one should embrace the opportunities to improve on existing capabilities within ourselves and acquire new abilities. If I fulfill a dream and reach my goal right away, a new dream and a new challenging goal are born and the desire to succeed and attain them pushes me forward. That's the secret of healing the body and mind: to become occupied with the things you like. Today, I can certainly say I made it! I recovered. I was able to realize the dreams I had. I continue to learn dancing and drawing, I read, cook, entertain, travel, and guide and advise others who wish to learn from my experience and more.

"All the situations in human life are required for man to perfect himself and the whole world and that is why no man will ever grow tired of the situation he is in, and act to fulfill his duties as it requires."
Rabi Kook

The anger inside me had apparently expressed my frustration at not being given an appropriate response about my condition. Everyone expresses his frustration in a different way. For the most part, it stems from childhood and how we survive in our primary family. This survival instinct provides protection and works well for children because it suits the conditions of childhood when we are helpless babies and children, entirely dependent on our parents for the satisfaction of our needs, security and love.

Everyone knows this and many psychological training methods were developed on this basis, treating people in order to cure them. This type of survival protected us in situations that made us feel pain, fear, threat, concern and distress. As children, it protected us, but as adults - as responsible and independent people with life experience, with capabilities and new skills that we have developed throughout our lives - we can choose our course of action, choose the reality we want to live in and work so that it will come true. The problem is that, as adults, we are often not connected to our independent abilities and to our mental energies, and still consider ourselves helpless, dependent and weak, which makes us insecure, fearful, ashamed, weak and lonely with lack of meaning and value. Accordingly, we act and behave and give our strengths to others, both close and distant, and expect them to protect us and keep us safe, to look after us and take care of us and save us from the pain caused by the helplessness.

When a need is not provided for us, we feel frustration and pain, in particular when we lose the ability to regulate our emotions and when we have no way to calm ourselves; when we do not know how to reduce the pressures and tensions that stir us up, it is then that frustration and pain turn to anger.

Anger sticks with us and it is hard to get rid of, especially when it is hidden.

Some people, who have a hard time expressing their frustration in a direct and assertive manner, express it in their old, familiar way: outbursts of rage toward those who were supposed to provide them with their need. Others will react according to their old habit and keep it inside, not express it at all and try to keep the relationship quiet, trying to be "okay" and please the other, but they feel anger inside and it will foster a sense of bitterness, discrimination, avoidance, lack of confidence, criticism, self-flagellation or depression. This festering may be reflected in all sorts of disease and other strange phenomena – fibromyalgia, possibly.

There are also those who, at first, try to contain the anger within them, but when they fail to do so, they end up bursting into a fury of rage and criticism towards those who left them (in their opinion) with lack of their needs. The outburst of anger is actually a cry of pain awakened within us, born out of an important and basic necessity left unsatisfied, especially when our expectation for fulfillment and satisfaction was from the people closest or most important to us. Thus, underlying the desire to be cured, one must first understand the supreme importance of easing the tensions and resentments we have accumulated and then find natural ways to neutralize, deconstruct and convert the anger into an expression of some sort of creativity. The process of creativity is the process of healing the wounded soul, no matter what reason brought us to this situation. Forgiveness provides balm to the injured soul; forgiveness neutralizes poisoned energies and allows soft reference and support to oneself, in the very one forgiving experiencing individual and had within hope and faith.

Stay away from bitterness. Step away from people who make you weak. Forgive those who make you uncomfortable and cover your anger with love. The best healing for the soul is to forgive and to do whatever pleases you and promotes your healthier, stronger, better life. Forgiveness does not change the past, but it allows the future to evolve and develop. The longer a person stays burrowed into his anger, the deeper it becomes etched in his consciousness so it is hard for him to break free. He is convinced that he is right, and an inner war rages within him, consuming his strength and impairing his judgment and reactions, thus increasing the chances of developing anxiety, fear, guilt and hardship. The ability to transform his life moves away from him.

Recovery involves change. At first, the change seems frightening and uncomfortable, and often it also involves risk.

Yet there seems to be no other way to build a healthier, better and happier life.

I paid dearly for the terrible anger, for the helplessness and frustration that I experienced in my life. I did not know how to channel them to a place that would lead me to be happy, joyous, healthy and creative and able to celebrate life with enjoyment.

I was afraid of losing what I had that was familiar. I avoided facing up to the things that were hard for me. Doubts and hesitations gnawed inside me day after day, until it became months and years and the flame extinguished. Today and every day, I thank the good Lord for watching over me and for the inner voice that cried within me for a change. A change that brought a better barter and profits, of hundred percents while transforming my life, from the profit I gained as a person with fibromyalgia syndrome.

Today, the key words of my life are balance, and listening to my body. I didn't stop being hypersensitive, on the contrary, but the negative phenomena that accompanied this sensitivity while I hadn't understood it ceased, the positive phenomena intensified, and I was able to channel this sensitivity into a rout that push my life forward in every way.

Happiness is Possible

Today, I stay safe for my own good and behave with awareness, foreseeing weakening or harmful moves and promoting measures that contribute to my health. I moderate or restrict myself out of joy, not out of victimhood or frustration. I am aware of myself, I value myself, I have confidence in myself. I love people and I transfer knowledge to others from my gained experience, from a place of awareness. Today, I am like everybody else: empathetic towards the person sitting in front of me. I understand him. I was there.

I learned on my own flesh and blood, and I counsel others now, that what is true for one is not necessarily true for the other. Release your judgment and self-criticism. Discover curiosity and lavish yourself with love, and results will soon follow. Give thanks for what you have and see all the good in you and around you. It gives power, strengthens the self-confidence and enhances love.

Know that when you act in your own best interests, you are going to experience life to the fullest and live in the moment and at the present from a place of natural pleasure and joy - joy that stems from the heart and does not depend on anything else.

The more gratitude I felt towards the things I have in my life, the more things there were to be thankful for... It is both surprising and

exciting and, of course, it provides tremendous motivation to continue onwards.

I slightly renovated my house and turned it into a gallery with proper lighting that emphasizes the beauty of my works. I welcome those who come to me from near and far, seeking guidance and counseling in the "Dos and Don'ts" that I developed to heal myself of the syndrome, and for meditation and guided imagery sessions.

My method grew out of personal experience, autodidactic self-study and by constantly striving for the desired result - optimal health. Largely, I redesigned my identity and also went through a professional transformation. From my new vantage point, which is complete and at peace, calm and full, and through deep insights and targeted questions, I banished the place of misery and introduced a place of acceptance, containment, forgiveness and compassion. The strong desire to share this knowledge with others was born, to support and help others promote themselves and to plant hope in their hearts by promoting the assumption that it is their right to change their lives and that the choice is theirs.

"In everyone's life, at some time, our inner fire goes out. It then bursts into flame due to an encounter with another human being. We should all be thankful for those people who rekindle the inner spirit."
Albert Schweitzer

I advise those who consult me on what they should do and must do to aid their recovery and what should they avoid, and to avoid activities that may harm their health. I also work with them to refine their decisions in life, and recommend being careful with prescriptions that were tried and tested for others, but may not work the same for us – the very hypersensitive people.

Moreover, you should ask yourself if the advice you've received is, indeed, suitable for who you are and for your particular case, whether you are comfortable with it or whether it's better to stand on your own because that will benefit you more. This advice is correct for any human being but more so for the hypersensitive person. Therefore, each person must develop his own personal seismograph, for his body, soul and ailments, until he sees the results that he wished for. If one way does not lead to the desired outcome, one has to think about changing direction, rethink and reevaluate, compare the gains and the losses for your mind and body and be willing to pay the price required for each action. Awareness at this level will set you free from unnecessary stress and unwanted surprises and if you do encounter them, you will know how to navigate yourself to the desired situation out of awareness and personal choice. You will know to repair, improve and 'tune up' better to decrease your level of suffering. We must aim to reduce every ailment that exists in the body or soul as much as possible, to the point of nonexistence.

This process requires self-commitment, goal setting, a certain level of consciousness and alertness, a strong desire, determination and dedication and all of the above must be bolstered by faith, compassion and great love for who you are, self-acceptance and a clear knowledge that you are perfect just as you are, and that you have the tools to change, improve, upgrade and achieve results and fulfill your dreams in good health.

The strength to defeat every darkness and make every sadness into great joy is to focus on the solutions and on what we want. This is a necessary condition to get what we want and create the reality that we hope for.

If there was a simple formula for success, or an easy magic trick to perform, most people would presumably use them to succeed.

I'm sure everyone reading this book can identify himself among its pages in some part, and maybe all of them. It's true that only someone who experienced the different sensations, can understand the suffering of others like him. This is why we should protect our feelings and insights as hyper sensitive people who are flooded with stimulations.

Sometimes we do not have the strength, the time or the ability to make a difference, but if we recognize the opportunity when it comes our way, grab it with both hands, embrace it and decide that it came for us and for our benefit, even if we do not have the necessary resources - strength, health, money, knowledge, education, help and more - we can always find within ourselves the spark that will light the fire, and from there the sky's the limit.

"When one door closes, another opens;
But we often continue to look
So regretfully at the closed door
That we do not see the one that opened before us."
(Alexander Graham Bell)

May this book inspire and give strength, open up a window in your heart, and awaken in you a spark and a flame of fire for a good, healthy, fulfilling and fun life. Energy flows where we turn our attention and the present is the moment of power. Recovery is possible and it is the right of every person to live with joy, happiness, good health and full realization of his life.

"Life is beautiful.
It is permitted to enjoy all its good.
Evrything is in the right order"
Nissim Amon - Israeli Zen Master

☐

Epilogue

I call to you, my reader:

If something of my story in this book spoke to you, write it down, embrace it in your heart. Copy it. Get out there and don't wait. In every direction you go, there are challenges. In every challenge, there are milestones until you get the result you want. The desired result is called success!

He who looks for health in magic tricks and free tips will discover that he is paying for them with his health and they will not solve his ills.

Do not allow any external factor to affect your life and mood. The life you experience today is the direct result of the choices you made or things you did not do in the past. Your choices are the ones that shape your reality and they are your responsibility.

Be who you are, know what you want and examine how you see yourself. Do you see yourself as you really are? Maybe you tend to underestimate yourself and your talent in front of others and even in front of yourself?

To truly be yourself means to stay true to yourself. Allow yourself to listen, consider and consult, but make the final decision by listening to your inner voice. Don't let anyone manipulate you. Keep control over whatever will deter you from your goals. Acknowledge who you are and be happy for it.

Don't wait for something to happen. Change your attitude and your actions and things will happen. Bring meaning and content to your life. Pain inside the body is a language one must learn to listen to, so do not ignore your body's cries - give them a proper response.

Collect information which is relevant to your condition. Do not let fate run your life. Bring zeal and diligence into your actions and results will soon follow. Change course if the solution is not in the path that you walk. Over time, learn to ask for help when you need it and share your troubles with your loved ones in order to create a brainstorming that will facilitate your recovery. Agree to be in a state of temporary uncertainty, take some time for deliberation and introspection. Get in touch with your true desire. Accept responsibility for change - there is no other but you who will do it for you. Identify the hardship and know that within it lies an opportunity for you, even if you do not see it in

88

your imagination at present. Live with gratitude - it is an important action for recovery. It's a way to see what is in life and to get strength.

People who want to get better understand the significance of the decision to recover, create the film of their lives and take responsibility for their recovery, while others believe that their lives depend on the doctors, on treatment, on pharmaceuticals and on circumstances that happen along the way.

There are only two choices and one chance: you either grow or you perish. What do you choose?

Find the right path for you. Give yourself back the power to take care of yourself, strengthen your self-belief and confidence in your abilities - for you were born with them. People who decide to recover, manage their health; the rest - their health manages them!

Add to all the above: softness, love and compassion towards yourself and the others.

**"If you ask me what I came into this life to do,
I will tell you: I came to live my life out loud!"
Émile Zola**

BOOKS THAT ACCOMPANIED THE ESSENTIAL PROCESS IN MY LIFE

Without Shortcuts - Smadar Ettinger

A woman in her own right - Rebecca Nardi

The Power of Your Subconscious Mind - Joseph Murphy

Child of the Dawn - Gautama Chopra

You Can Heal Your Life - Louise L. Hay

Don't Sweat the Small Stuff - Richard Carlson

Mutant Message Down Under - Marlo Morgan

Your Erroneous Zones - Dr. Wayne Dyer

The Power of Intention - Dr. Wayne Dyer

Between Despair and Hope - Mordechai Krup

The Monk Who Sold His Ferrari - Robin S. Sharma

The Saint, the Surfer, and the CEO - Robin S. Sharma

Who Will Cry When You Die? - Robin S. Sharma

A Friendly Change - Rafi Yaakoby

The Artist's Way: A Spiritual Path to Higher Creativity - Julia Cameron

The Artist's Way at Work: Riding the Dragon - Julia Cameron

When Things Fall Apart - Pema Chodron

The Man Who Managed to Change the Film - Rafael Hacohen

Awekning to Life - Ronit Doron

The New Earth - Eckhart Tolle

A Moment Before the Psychiatrist - Dr. Pinky Feinstein

The Highly Sensitive Person - Dr. Elaine Aron

Talor Sela

ABOUT THE AUTHOR

Talor Sela, daughter of Holocaust survivors, a mother of four boys, is now a counselor and alternative therapies consultant, lecturer, an intuitive painter and hosts workshops for meditation and guided imagination.

www.fibromialgia.co.il
talorsela@gmail.com

www.ingramcontent.com/pod-product-compliance
Lightning Source LLC
Chambersburg PA
CBHW050420290526
45786CB00003B/1341